ANGELS
UNDER MY BED

Carol Ann Creagh

The White Row Press

*With thanks to the dedicated consultants and staff
at the Cancer Centre, Belfast City Hospital,
for your care and your caring on my journey*

ANGELS
UNDER MY BED

Carol Ann Creagh

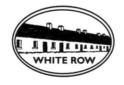

The White Row Press

First published 2011
by the White Row Press Ltd.
135 Cumberland Road, Dundonald
Belfast BT16 2BB

Front cover photograph: Carol Ann Creagh
Back cover: (L-R) Grandpop, Carol Ann aged four,
Carol Ann with her 'string of pearls', Philip and Carol Ann in the hospice

Cover design: Cheah
Typesetting: Island Publications
Printed by the Gutenberg Press, Malta

A catalogue record for this book is available from the British Library

ISBN 978 1 870132 41 1

Contents

Preface

Cancer sneaks up on you
While you are asleep
And then your life is changed...

June 2006, as dawn was breaking outside our beautiful home where my beautiful family slept, I cried inconsolably as I wrote the first lines of the poem that began this story. Four years had passed since my breast cancer diagnosis and I was falling apart, physically, mentally and emotionally. Unhappiness was overwhelming me as I screamed silent screams.

Waking at 4 am that morning something told me the voice inside me needed to speak.

Armed with a file block from one of my kid's desks I sat in the cool, early morning sun and wrote. Words not taken from my head or my hand but from my heart spilled over every page. I had found my healing route. Weeks would pass as chapter after chapter was written on top of marshmallow beds in Ballycastle, or at McArts Fort high on the Cavehill. When it was written I slipped it into my memory box under the bed.

June 2010, a girlie day out with Big Sis, Janet and another friend would make me eventually reopen that box again. Up the Antrim coast, somewhere between greasy chips and candy floss, we had an Angel card reading. Wiping my fingers free of sticky, pink sugar, I picked my cards, lay them on the dark, cloth-covered table, and listened to their message:

Your angels have been telling you for five years to write your story.

Later, over a few white wines we all recounted the light hearted tales of our cards. Laughing I dismissed the very thought of writing a book. I'm not a writer. My 1 in English Literature at O Level was an appreciation of other writers' work. My 4 in English Language was the best I could achieve for my own. My story stayed under the bed.

Well, until one winter's day when I returned from yet another abnormal scan. Crawling under my bed and opening my memory box I pulled the many handwritten pages out from where they nestled between hospital baby bracelets and handmade Mother's Day cards. Maybe I needed to write this story for my six children, my string of pearls. If some day, I was to lose my fight with cancer, I needed them to remember me. Remember their "wee mummy" who loved them so much and would miss them forever...

And if my story, my journey helps even one person newly diagnosed with cancer, then it was worth writing.

For my wonderful dad who now sleeps with his angels

1

I hope all dogs go to heaven

March the 17th blurred into itself. I came back home from my friend Claire's to the madness of St. Paddy's Day. The three girls were planning a few bevvies in the house and then a party somewhere. My three boys, still too young, were champing at the bit to do something. Me, I just wanted to run to the Antrim coast, where the winds would clear my head and the waves battering the spring coastline would somehow give me the strength I needed to face the next week. Who was I kidding? It wasn't strength I needed, it was a bloody miracle.

An hour earlier, with her GP hat on, Claire had poked and prodded me while I lay rigid on her duvet, and insisted that 90% of breast lumps were benign. I agreed! We were both too scared to mention the big C word, but it was there like an elephant sitting on the end of the bed.

The woes of the day didn't end there. I arrived back to find the girls in pieces. Our little white Westie, Charlie, had got out with all the coming and going. He'd made it to the top of the road where he had been hit by a passing bus. His little, limp body lay on the kitchen floor, his head resting on Emma's lap. It was too much. My eyes gave way to the tears I'd been holding back all day. The grim reaper had visited our house that day and was determined to take someone out of it. Maybe wee Charlie was looking out for me and he went instead. My tears rolled onto his soft fur, the children's tears could not be stopped. I had no words to make it better. We buried him the next day and my silent prayer was, 'I hope all dogs go to heaven'.

Bank holiday Monday over, Claire kicked into action, calling in a few favours. On Wednesday at 8.30 am my fate would be decided. Twenty-three hours and twenty-two minutes left of normality. At 8 am that Wednesday, the City Hospital looked no different from usual. Shifts of day nurses reporting for duty, and weary night nurses heading to their cars for a cosy sleep under their duvets on this bitterly cold March day. I looked up at the thirteenth floor of the Nurses' Home, counted three windows across and saw my home of three years. The place I'd lived, loved and laughed in as a seventeen year old was about to turn on me.

I loved that six by eight foot room with its bird's eye view of Belfast and my Cavehill in the distance. I could still see the bed in the corner, the under-drawers stuffed to bursting point with my blue-check student uniforms, starched aprons and stiff collars. Cuffs didn't frequent those drawers too often as I usually lost them a week after I bought them, while the elusive studs – two for your belt and one for your collar – changed hands outside the lifts between those going on and those coming off duty. It was a frantic scramble when we were all doing the same shifts. For your uniform had to be just so. To be seen without any part of it, even the smallest stud, came close to being a sackable offence – or so we thought. My favourite piece was the big, wool, navy cape with its bright red lining. If you were on night duty and headed over to the Nurses' Home for your midnight lunch when the nurses' disco was on, it always assured you of a dance. In fact, come to think of it, I got more dances in my uniform than out of it.

Off duty, my built-in wardrobe was used as a swap shop for any size eight to ten nurse. A few size twelves tried and failed, and anyone over five foot one didn't stand a chance. The desk to the right of the window was filled with knick-knacks and memorabilia of nights out with the boys I'd loved and lost and the boys I'd loved and left, while family pictures and soft toys weighed down the shelf above. And of course, a little space was left for studying, but that was mainly done in bed curled up in my oversized pj's and fluffy socks. Abba's Dancing Queen playing loudly on my cherished record player warmed us all up for the disco, and a bit of Roxy Music, Bread or David Cassidy (Could it be Forever – swoon!) saw us through the post mortem in the wee small hours. And for my best friend Rosie, I'd throw in a bit of country & western. Painful I know, but it had to be done for her.

Yes, in that room I fell in and out of love many, many times. I nursed many a hangover from experimenting with Pernod and blackcurrant, whiskey and blackcurrant (wouldn't recommend it), and cider and blackcurrant. The only part of my tipples that never changed was the blackcurrant. Not so good though, second time round when my head was chucking it up over the sink. Yes, this was the place that prepared me for adulthood, but was this to be the place that would now cut that adulthood short? Had I laughed too much, was it now the time for tears?

I took my eyes away from the thirteenth floor of my past

and looked to the hospital's massive tower block – the block which held the people and machines that would now decide my future. Not a scary building, in fact the foyer with its shop and coffee corner had quite a friendly buzz about it. A short walk took me towards the first signpost of my journey: Outpatients.

2

Why me? Why not me?

Timidly, I went to the desk, stated my name and address, then Patrick and I took our seats among a scattering of women. It was only 8.20 am, so there were plenty of seats to choose from.

Eyes rose to look in my direction, maybe because I had that 'new kid on the block' look, or maybe it was because I still had a full head of hair, a tell-tale sign that this was my first visit. They were sympathetic glances, empathetic glances. All girls together.

Name called, I walked calmly to the room behind the nurse. My heart was pumping in my chest, my head, even my limbs – could she hear it? I felt nausea well up from the pit of my gut, but no breakfast assured that it remained in place. When the consultant spoke to me I could hardly get my tongue off the roof of my mouth. But somehow I kept it together, giving her a big smile and mumbling a few words about what I'd found. Her manner was brisk and efficient, even verging on cold. But that was OK as one ounce of sympathy and I'd have lost it. Note taking, examination, and a needle stuck into my left boob over, I was sent outside to wait three hours on the lab report.

'Come back at twelve,' they said, handing my fate, on a three inch slide, to a faceless technician, a man or maybe a woman who probably wouldn't even get round to it till after their tea-break. After all, who was I? Just a faceless name on a lab request. Not really a person, a mother, a wife, a daughter, a sister, a friend. No, I was just a few cells smeared on a little piece of glass. As a nurse, I sent a hundred samples to the lab every day, kidding myself that I was empathetic to all these patients... boy, I didn't even come close.

Three hours isn't usually very long. In my day I could have filled it ten times over, but that day someone stopped my watch and every clock within a five-mile radius. Every minute seemed like an hour and every hour seemed like an eternity. I had time to play out in my head all my reactions. Good news! That would be the easy one. But bad news, now that proved a little bit tougher to write the script for, as I didn't have an ending. Really bad news... well, best not go there!

The scene was set when I returned to Outpatients. We were the only two there. Oh no! Not a good sign. Keep bad news and tears away from an audience. The nurse walked past me and went for back up. The cancer specialist nurse. Oh no. I had played this scene so often as a senior casualty nurse that I knew the script backwards. I left Patrick in the waiting room and took the ten steps required to reach my future, or lack of it. Funny, I felt strangely calm, void of emotions, numb... I mean, how bad could it be? I was a fit, healthy forty-four year old. I could get through this. Couldn't I?

Malignant!

Benign: that's a little, fat, cute cell. Something you could live with, something you could be attached to forever, a friendly lump. But no, my lump wasn't to be fat, round and cosy. It was harsh, jagged and aggressive, a bad cell growing inside me. A malignancy! Spreading its evil around my body through the breasts that fed my babies, the small size 32b that made me feel like a woman. The breasts that could now kill me.

I listened calmly as a plan was arranged. The two nurses kept guard, ready to pounce on my reaction, but I was trained for this. Well, maybe not for this side of the desk, but I wanted to remain composed so I kept listening. It is true though, what they say about patients only hearing one third of what you tell them. I left the room with two thirds bouncing off the consulting room walls and ceiling. Malignant! I really didn't need to hear anymore!

Out in the waiting room I calmly told Patrick it wasn't good news and from that moment on our paths began to separate. Not obvious at first, but the seed had been planted. A slow, insidious silence grew between us. Words didn't get spoken. We were both trying to go in the same direction, but we read the map differently and began to veer apart.

In the safety of the car silent tears rolled down my cheeks as I watched the Nurses' Home fade into the distance, taking with it all my hopes and dreams. Yes, maybe I had laughed too much and it was now the time for tears. So I let them fall gently down my cheeks because I knew that when I reached home I would have to dig deep, hide my tears, and put on a brave face. I had ten minutes to cry my heart out. Just ten minutes.

Up to this point only three people had known about my check up: Patrick, Claire and my eldest daughter Sam, as damage limitation would be easier that way – there was no point in causing unnecessary worry. But now the family jungle drums beat overtime. The doorbell never stopped. The kettle never cooled and the phone never ceased. It was all very strange. It was like being at my own wake. Family had tears in their eyes, people were starting to have masses said, candles were being lit, and I was being given every relic known to man.

Why?

I looked well. I felt well. Yet, bizarrely, I might be dying! My eyes welled up every so often but I continued to smile. Yes, it's easy to smile from your lips but it's not so easy to smile from your eyes. If I avoided eye contact no one would see my despair. I talked positive to everyone, quoting stories of all the survivors I knew, it was safer not to think of those who hadn't. I knew what had to be done. If anyone in our family had to go through this, I was probably a good choice. I might be the smallest in size but I made up for that in feistiness. I am strong and I would fight it all the way.

With the exception of the maternity ward I had never been on the patient's side of the bed. I had always prided myself on my good health. I ate healthy, never smoked, and as for alcohol, two drinks and I was pickled. I also loved exercise. Walking, cycling, jogging, gym workouts – you name it, I enjoyed it. Now I prayed that this would get me through what lay ahead.

Cancer. Why do people get it? I don't think anyone can really answer that question. It's a word many find difficult to say. It's often spoken in a hushed, reverential whisper under the breath. To say it out loud makes it real. And the reality is – cancer kills. Is cancer a punishment for something done in your youth? Is it a cruel, character building exercise? Or maybe it's caused by the stresses of life sending your body's defences crashing down around you.

Why me?

Well, why not me?

3

Matters of love and money

M other to six, wife to one, nurse practitioner to 8,200. Hard to keep those balls all in the air, and then of course there was the money pit! A monster house in a grand, tree-lined avenue. A street inhabited by the wealthy of the world. So what were we doing there? Yes, we could afford to buy it. It was a tip which no one else wanted. Of course we could buy it. The estate agents were glad to see some idiots take it off their hands. Even the surveyor said, 'Take my advice, buy a house round the corner.' But we believed we could sort it. On a teacher's and a nurse's salary – don't make me laugh! We were at least two pay packets short. And every builder that opened our leafy suburban gate saw pound signs. As they came down the path, the quotes rose with every step they took. By the time I opened the front door there were more zeros in their estimates than in a tin of spaghetti hoops. Big house doesn't always mean big wage. In our case it just meant big family.

After many a sharp intake of breath, each builder inhaling more deeply than the last – for the task that faced them was truly daunting – the repair work finally started. A living, eating, breathing programme – living in dirt and squalor. Eating takeaways as we often had no electricity or running water, and breathing in dust from kangos and plaster. Getting ourselves to work and the kids to school was the bonus of the day, as there was heat, food and water to be had in those places. My lunch breaks though, were often spent in builders' yards. I went so often all the sales staff got to know me, probably because I stood out like a sore thumb in my navy sister's uniform. But night times were the worst. I didn't get to rest. When the madness of the day died down, I had to take myself up to a cold attic room and, wrapped in scarf and woolly jumper, type up the assignments for my nurse practitioner degree.

Yes, this house was a millstone round our necks. It would take us to hell and back. But hell might have been better – at least it would have been warm there!

Money was getting very tight, builders needed paying and we couldn't earn it as fast as we could spend it. The Monster's financial arteries were haemorrhaging. So we embarked on major surgery. In '93 we had bought a lovely little terrace house in the country, but in October '97 it had to be amputated to save the Monster. Its mortgage would free up our capital, and the money from the sale would pay the builders.

We were sorry to have to get rid of it. It was an idyllic little place. Estate agents were tripping over themselves to get it on their books, and it soon attracted a keen buyer. But by December everything had changed. In December the deeds were read. Our living room was owned by the house next door and we had no right-of-way to our garage! A blind man could see it on the deeds. What did we pay a solicitor for in '93? Did he even bother to look at the damn things? Our house was being handed out to the district piece by piece, and it didn't take long for this juicy bit of gossip to spread through the village and surrounding countryside. Sitting on the stairs at 4.20 pm on the 8th December 1997, I received a phone call informing us that the buyer had pulled out, just an hour before completion. Completely numb, I put down the phone. I looked at the builders working all round me. How on earth were we going to pay them?

We had reached the gates of hell and spent the next five years up to our necks in a legal swamp, trying to reason with solicitors, estate agents, the law society and potential buyers.

*

What could we do? The Monster was guzzling money, the country retreat was unsellable. My attempted solution was to take three jobs. My original one, as a nurse practitioner, Monday to Thursday, then moonlighting in a second GP practice on a Friday, and agency nursing back in my old stomping ground, Casualty in the Mater Hospital, most Saturdays and Sundays.

So, nineteen years after I'd started my first shift as an inexperienced, young staff nurse, I made my way back to the Mater. The memories flooded back. On Mayday, 1980, as a naïve twenty-one year old, I had entered the Mater with great trepidation, pushing open its heavy double doors, and walking into its large, square waiting-room, not knowing what would greet me. My last visit had been as a very young child and it hadn't changed a bit. The building, hewn into the prison next door, had a beautiful, terrazzo floor and a grey, perspex roof, with three review cubicles to the left, one used as a sister's office, and a large Casualty Theatre directly ahead. Through the high windows you could see people's ankles passing by. So not only was it built into a wall, it must have been built into a hole.

The place still had the same strong, clean smell: hibiscrub, savlon and carbolic, which evoked childhood memories of getting my little finger stitched back together. It was an old building, very old, but it was immaculate, courtesy of Mrs Brown who took great pride in cleaning her little corner of the health service. Germs didn't stand a chance. So clean was it, that if my egg bap hit the deck I could safely eat it on retrieval... I didn't, but I could have.

These were the famous egg baps ordered at 8 am from Maggie's hatch, a hut-like box to the rear of the waiting room. We didn't need to go to the canteen when Maggie was there to create her delights. Everything prepared each day from scratch had nurses, doctors, ambulance staff and patients alike fighting for her last sandwich. Those of us lucky enough to be her favourites had ours secreted under the counter till the hunger pangs of lunchtime arrived.

To the right of this busy hatch, Tom's wheelchairs stood to attention. Cleaned and counted daily, their black, shiny, vinyl seats were ready to escort the immobile to their bedsides. Woe betide if you took one to the ward and came back without it, as it took quite a lot of grovelling and cajoling to get back into his good books.

Andy and Mac ran the plaster room, a white gypsona-filled space to the other side of the hatch. A place where I would spend many winters, arms up to my elbows in blood-temperature water. Too hot or too cold, the plaster hardened too quickly. There was a just right somewhere in between. I prided myself on my short leg, long leg, short arm, long arm, scaphoid pop (plaster of Paris) masterpieces. But the proof was passing Andy's and Mac's eagle eyes. A nod from them and you were well on the way to your prize: a big, cream bun bought from the bakery nearby. Creamy plaster and creamy buns, it was a great room to spend a shift in on a frosty winter's day.

The Mater itself was an old hospital built with wards in two turrets and an Intensive Care Unit (ICU), theatres and X-ray unit trapped somewhere in between; and of course, the little chapel around which each day revolved. Sundays were always good, and a mass break even for non-Catholics, assured everyone of a long tea-break, which was even more welcome if it followed a heavy Saturday night out. This break was a tradition set by the nuns, who had run the hospital since it opened. It was only taken over by the health service as recently as the seventies, on the understanding that a nun would be the matron. Her task of steering this ship was not made easy as it lay in volatile waters. A staunchly loyalist area lay to its front, a nationalist one to its rear, both meeting in Casualty where, on a regular basis, fighting spilled out over Mrs Brown's spotless, terrazzo floor.

I spent six of my later years there on night duty, fending off many a fracas with the help of the over-used panic button. This would bring the boys in blue. But often their arrival would only escalate the problem. Bottles and even wheelchairs would go soaring through the air, clanking into trolleys with no regard for the heart-attack patients who lay on them, watching the black pantomime unfold.

Fuelled by too much drink, these fracas could last into the

small hours of the morning. The waiting room only emptied as admissions were safely dispatched to a warm bed in a quiet ward, discharges got sent home to cold beds, or maybe escorted to a hard bed over the wall in the Crumlin Road Prison, where they could nurse their hangovers.

Of course, it wasn't all high drama. My early years in the hospital were filled with fun. We were all twenty-something staff nurses trying to become sisters; and young housemen, wet behind the ears from university, full of their own importance, all set to cure the world from the little yellow 'Bible' tucked in their white, starched coat pockets.

It was a volatile cocktail. Love and romance were often in the air. But I was exempt from all of this as I had arrived with a ring on my finger. So I watched from the wings. Long hours and hard work were mixed with loads of laughter, tinged with black humour. Saturday afternoons were a popular shift. The waiting room walls and chairs were lined with big, strapping sportsmen, brought down by dirty tackles. And when a five foot nurse applied a figure of eight to their fractured clavicles, more often than not these six foot forwards would hit the deck for a second time.

Being chatted up went with the territory. I got some very sweet and some downright blushful chat-up lines. But it was all innocent fun as I was out of bounds. Or at least I was, until Jim the new houseman arrived. Every time we shared a shift my cheeks would pink up till they glowed crimson. Trying to stop it mid-flight was not an option. He had a girlfriend, I had a fiancée, but that didn't stop my heart thumping when I as much as caught a glimpse of him. I kept it under control for five months but then

Christmas came and with it the Christmas party.

We talked into the small hours, perched on the windowsill till the dawn was breaking. I was head over heels about him and I'd a diamond ring on my finger. This wasn't good. I told Patrick I was worried I was falling for someone. He laughed it off. So I muddled through most of January with my feelings intact but a second work's night out was to be a disaster. Jim drove me home, said he would leave his girlfriend and now it was up to me. I was the one with the ring on my finger. The ball was in my court. But I didn't know where to hit it. I was falling in love with this person but to be with him I would have to hurt another. And I didn't know if I could do that. Next day, when my shift finished, Patrick called for me. I told him what had happened and within minutes he was hammering on the doctor's door. Thankfully, there was no reply. So instead he revved up his car, taking off at speed with my leg and the passenger door flying in the wind. Dumping me outside my home, he sped off down the road before I could say anything.

I was a free woman. Not quite in the way I'd planned, but then things never really go the way you plan. I started dating Jim, but I had destroyed a person and bad karma was on its way. After only two months, when I was away on a week's holiday, Jim two-timed me with a housewoman, a far better prize than a nurse. The circle of hurt was complete. I'd given up everything for him and I'd hurt another person in the process, yet it seemed to count for nothing to him. My shifts were changed to avoid Jim and his new girlfriend, the pain easing with each day. I licked my wounds and life went on. In time, Patrick came back, but the ring stayed in the box. Maybe being engaged at twenty was not to be recommended, so we decided to wait and start dating again. I never saw Jim again after that day and life went on in Casualty. New housemen, new romances came and went, but I remained safely tucked in the wings.

Life in Accident and Emergency wasn't all laughter and romance. There were many sad, dark days in the eighties when death visited our Casualty through bombs and guns. Young men, often boys, arrived clinging to life. And we were unable to save them. Youngsters reduced to corpses for a distraught mother or father to identify.

But at least these sons were still recognisable. It was not so easy preparing a bomb victim. On one occasion, I couldn't make out a boy's face to clean him up before his mum came in to see what was left of the child she had raised, only to be annihilated before his adult life had properly begun. On another, I attended a mother whose son was shot and whose husband, on hearing the news, took a heart attack. Both lay dead side-by-side in Casualty Theatre. I took her behind the curtain to say her goodbyes. I had no words to take away her pain so I just held her hand. Ten minutes later I watched her go home to an empty house to arrange a double funeral.

In 1991, I left the world I had loved for eleven years. I had grown weary of being so close to death and destruction, not only from the troubles – cot deaths, road traffic accidents, drownings and fires – it had all got too much. I could no longer cope. But now the time had come to return. A new millennium, a new Casualty building, a new staff. Lots had changed since I had packed up my fob watch. E.R., Casualty, and technology had taken over this world. Green scrubs confused staff and public alike as to who was who in the health chain. Gone was the old building, Mrs Brown's pristine terrazzo floor, and Martin's trolleys. Maggie's food hatch had been replaced by a vending machine. But saddest of all, the heartbeat of the old Casualty was missing.

Mrs Stewart our senior sister, our mother-figure, our confidante, our hug in dark days, had left a year earlier due to ill health. Her office, once filled with rotas, order books, and half-drunk cups of coffee, had fallen silent. This was where we had Christmas parties, hen parties and leaving parties. Where sausage rolls and curled up ham sandwiches filled her desk to be quickly scoffed between suturing and sorting. Where there were tissue stacks in the corner for the relatives who wouldn't be taking their loved ones home. A son, a daughter, a mother, a father a baby, a tragedy, she always had a supporting arm for them and the right words to say. And on the back of the door a change of uniform for when blood splatterings could not be avoided.

But now those navy dresses and frilly starched hats were gone and in their place a more practical garb of trousers and clogs had arrived. As had a world of league tables and waiting times. But alphabetically graded nurses could not replace this large, warm, lovable sister who gave thirty years to nurturing and caring for the people of north Belfast. Now, as I stood in my agency uniform of navy trousers and white tunic surrounded by a technological minefield of machines and tubes, I ached a little for what once was. I didn't want to be here without her and Mrs Brown, and Maggie and Sammy, but I had bills to pay. I didn't have a choice.

4

Falling apart

My life as I knew it was un-ravelling. Running three jobs, home life, cooking and cleaning in what hours were left, I was drowning, and nobody was chucking me a lifebelt. Maybe I should have spoken up but for whatever reason, while I was screaming inside, it never reached my vocal cords. I think I hoped someone would notice I was sinking and save me, but maybe they thought I was waving not drowning.

I juggled my way through 2000 pretty well. Tending towards Obsessive Compulsive Disorder, I had a routine, and if I stuck to it, I could get through the week. Things even began to look up. By the summer there was a glimmer of light at the end of the tunnel when someone asked if they could rent the little house. Yes, money! A monthly income until the deeds got sorted... or so I thought.

We drove down, met our tenant, got a guarantor and handed her the key. In six months she paid three rents, no deposit, destroyed our home, and sent us a solicitor's letter because we had dared to suggest that she wasn't maintaining it. Another damn solicitor!

We had made this discovery by chance. My brother and I had gone down in October to leave the woman in some wallpaper.

When she opened the door we were met by a terrible stench. Her young children were running around toileting where they wanted. Three huge dogs were doing the same. Our carpets and furniture were ruined. The children were sleeping on bare mattresses. Our little home had been turned into a rat-infested, foul smelling squat. I gently told her the place had to be cleaned or I would terminate the agreement (gently because I was afraid she'd change the locks!), and then cried all the way home in my brother's car. Her response was to go to a solicitor. So we gave her three months' notice.

In mid-January I drove down with knots in my gut for fear I'd be locked out, but she was out on the street, bags packed, waiting for a social services taxi to ferry her and her brood to their next poor victim's home, twenty miles away. When I walked through the house I felt physically sick from the sights and smells that greeted me. How could anyone live like that? How could they do this to someone's property? Mountains of rubbish lay against the wall of my lean-to. Rat droppings, stale food, and decomposing nappies were scattered throughout the house and garden. I didn't know if I could tackle this. A decontamination team would have had difficulty coping with the filth they left.

Half-suffocated, I stepped outside the front door gasping for fresh air. A lad in his twenties pulled up on his bike, and asked if the house was for rent. I told him there was no way I could rent it to man or beast in its present state. He came through it with me and said he would help me clean it out. Had God sent me an angel? That day I think he had.

For nine hours, the two of us worked tirelessly, scrubbing

walls, carpets and furniture, escaping every so often to the garden for fresh air. Each room brought more misery and filth, but nothing prepared either of us for the visit to the garage. She had locked her dog into a rabbit hutch and it had eaten its own leg out of hunger. What kind of person was she? Photos were taken and the NSPCA went after her, but she never turned up in court.

After the day we had gone through, I could think of nothing better than renting the house to this lovely lad. It was the least I could do. So, deposit swapped and hands shaken, I drove to my parents' nearby cottage where I stood in the shower for an hour, trying to rid myself of the foul smells, but they remained in my nostrils all night.

In the morning Patrick arrived down. Given the disaster experienced with our first tenant, he said we wouldn't be renting to anyone again and I had to give the deposit back. So, shame-faced and with much regret, I returned the cash to this lad who had been my angel of mercy,

I was now in free fall. It was 2001 and I was having chest pains and my pulse, which should have been just 78, was registering 178. I wasn't feeling well. After an ECG, Claire sent me to the chest pain clinic. The diagnosis was arrhythmias caused by stress burnout. I was told to take things easy – but how? Inside, my voice was screaming for help, but outside, it was silent. So I just got on with things, standing half asleep in the shower at 6.30 am most Saturdays and Sundays, getting ready for another thirteen hour shift in Casualty.

In the end my dad and brother bought the little house from us, but by then the debts were mountainous, so the two and three jobs continued. I hadn't heeded the warning. I didn't feel I could afford to. I had to keep going. But at 11.30 pm on 16th March 2002, I had no option. Everything came to a standstill. I felt a lump.

5

Silence

Looking back, I don't know why my voice remained silent. Most people who know me see me as a bubbly, extroverted person. So what was it that kept the words that I needed to speak trapped in my body, too deep for even me to reach?

My earliest memory of keeping silent was when, at the age of five years, I was in the back seat of a car and an adult put the seat down on my foot and sat on it. I didn't scream. I don't know why not. But I whispered to my sister what had happened and her yell nearly crashed the car. My little foot was black for days.

Maybe it was because we were brought up on the philosophy that 'children should be seen and not heard'. A large family, we were raised firmly but fairly, not unusual for the sixties. Or maybe it was too many years of nuns beating you into silence. In their book, noise deserved punishment.

Twenty-five years of my life, from the tender age of four, were lived according to nuns' rules. My first encounter fooled me. Sister Anthony was a beautiful nun, an angel who glided around the room in her habit. Nuns never had feet or hair. Any hint of womanhood was protected by yards and yards of heavy, black material held together by a dark, leather belt and a large, chunky rosary. Faces were tightly framed in white, starched headgear to which was attached a large, heavy veil. Scary to the average four year old, but not on Sister Anthony. She was different. And she had the sweetest, softest voice.

She loved all her Primary Ones. She would give us little treats from her tin for being good, or for bringing in our penny for the black babies. Those big, copper pennies that stained your hand green could have bought two half-penny chews in the tuck shop. But they were sent to faraway places to buy black babies half-penny chews instead. I loved giving in that big, smelly penny. Sister Anthony's only crime was to chastise me for trying to write with my crayon in my mitted hand. For whatever reason, left-handedness was frowned upon, and it was seen as an act of kindness to force you to write with your right hand. This is why they put mittens on our left hands. But they did so in vain. It never worked !

The safety and innocence of Primary One was to end abruptly. The Sisters of Mercy would show me no mercy for the next three years of my life, with each successive nun outdoing her predecessor. As we got bigger, so too did the punishments. Most of these were dished out with a sadism incomprehensible to five year olds. Thick wood would lash across tiny hands and wrists for little or no reason. Forgetting your lunch money, missing a word while reading, or for not standing in a straight line. These were hardly crimes, but in the sixties it was seen as acceptable for nuns, priests and brothers to dish out corporal punishment without question, to make us good, strong Christians... but we were only babies.

In Primary Three the nun was older, so her punishments

came from a seated position. A large hand lashing the back of your legs often sent you tumbling to the floor. Through the P2 and P3 years I was often physically sick on the way to school, crying in the car, begging my dad to take me home. He would take me to the door, explain to a very sweet nun how I was feeling, and then when he left, I got blattered.

But this was nothing compared to the evil that lay in wait for us in P4. This nun was so cruel that I started wetting the bed out of sheer terror. Her punishment was daily and harsh, and meted out to the entire class. The innocent were treated no different from the guilty. We all had to stand around the walls while she went round every hand with a large, thick, wooden stick. Pull it away and you could be assured of a second whack. Friday, 'tables' day, was by far the worst. My palms were red and hot with terror before I was asked any question, and redder and hotter still afterwards with the pain.

Whatever made these women become nuns? Were they forced into a life they hated? And were poor, defenceless children an easy target on which to vent their anger? No one stopped them. They owned the school. They made the rules. Parents accepted this without question, it was the way things were. But that didn't make it right. These full-grown women terrorized children, and no one did a thing.

Was this the beginning of my silence? Fear and subservience was what we learnt. If someone said jump, you would ask how high. It was never your place to challenge, you put up and shut up. We grew into young adults trying to please, keeping the peace and never pushing the boundaries. These were the qualities or afflictions I carried into my marriage and my career. In nursing,

I worked twice as hard to prove my family life would not get in the way of doing my job. At home I'd over-compensate for being a working mother. The guilt of leaving my own children while I went to look after other people's never sat well with me. But what could I do? The second salary was a necessity not a luxury.

My solution was to invent a version of The Little House on the Prairie and place it at the foot of Walton Mountain. Delegating didn't exist. The little voice stayed silent. Trying to create perfection in all aspects of your life is impossible and I was about to pay the price. Cancer was about to bring Walton Mountain crashing down around me. I was knackered. I had breast cancer. Now I needed to dig deep inside myself and come out fighting for myself. Up until this point, I'd been a fighter for every cause known to man. I'd walked in peace rallies, anti-war protests. Give me an injustice and I'd lead from the front. But my own fight? Now that was a different story. I'd hoped someone would step up for me. But if you act like you're in control and coping, why would anyone do that? Being strong day in day out was something I'd spent years perfecting. But cancer was to challenge this to the core. Would I be strong enough to control it, or would it control me? I was about to enter the unknown.

6

The waiting is the worst

Oncology is a department within the great National Health Service which no one knows much about. A secret sect which operates from behind iron-lined walls and uses toxic drugs which would have the rest of the profession running for cover. Yet, when you enter this world you feel safe in their care. They know what they're doing. They work as a team, and take you by the hand through the cancer minefield.

Within days of diagnosis my admission was arranged. My surgery would be on Good Friday – not a bad day to carry a cross. Patrick and one of my sons left me over to the ward. My son John was oblivious to what was happening. Like any twelve year old, he just wanted to play with all the gadgets attached to the bed while I chatted to him about how we'd make ourselves sick on too many Easter eggs. As he charged out through the double doors, my heart cracked easier than any egg.

Looking around, I saw I wasn't alone. I was in a six-bedded unit, all of us sharing a common bond. Tomorrow we would part with a little piece of our womanhood, motherhood, body. A lovely lady across the ward adopted me as the baby of the gang. She was so taken with my pyjamas she sent her husband out to get her a pair.

Surgery knocked me for six. I was the first on the list but the last to wake up. Drugs and I don't gel very well. But by the next day I was able to wobble to the shower, remove my dressing rather sheepishly and feel pleasantly surprised by how much of me was left. Partial mastectomies were the preferred surgery to preserve womanhood. My lump was near the tail, a small piece of breast near the armpit, so my scar wasn't too bad. My left arm was numb to the elbow (a side-effect that has never left me – but a small price to pay), and I had a little hole under my armpit for a drain. All in all a neat, wee job and at least the cancer was no longer growing inside me. Instead it was lying in a histopathology bucket awaiting examination which would determine my fate. Would I be given the death sentence or would I be given a reprieve? The waiting is the worst. No matter how far you run, you can't escape your mind.

Discharged from hospital and not really up to it, I ran with the kids to Counties Fermanagh, Down and Antrim. I was exhausted, but if I stood still my mind would do the running for me. Monday arrived and I could run no further. This was the day of reckoning. The day I was to go back to hospital to hear what the removed lump contained. What made it worse was that it was a beautiful, fresh, April morning. Trees and flowers were starting to bud. Colour was coming into the garden. Spring was blooming all around me on the day my blooming might stop.

The ward floor felt like toffee and my feet sank with each step I took towards the consultant's office. This time I couldn't read their faces. No smiles, no frowns. In front of them a small piece of paper sat on top of a thin chart. Upside down it was indecipherable. The consultant shook my hand and at that moment I felt sorry for him. His was not an easy job. How could he have enjoyed his scone and coffee up in the staff canteen twenty minutes earlier knowing fine well he was going to give me news that would change or possibly end my life? I smiled at him to help make it easier. If it had been the fifteenth century and he was the axe man about to behead me, I possibly would have crossed his palm with silver too, but this was 10.30 am on 8th April, 2002. The smile had to do.

'I have some good news and some bad news.'

Good sounds good! Let's have that one first. It hadn't spread yet. OK, that's the bonus ball sorted, now what's the bad?

'It's an aggressive Grade 3, Her2 positive, oestrogen receptor negative, with a high risk of spread.'

Now I knew why he said, 'hadn't spread yet'.

So, aggressive therapy was needed for this bad boy: eight chemotherapy and twenty-five radiotherapy sessions, X-rays, bone scans, body scans, blood tests... my boobs were about to be viewed by more people than if I'd put them on page three of the Sun. Well, that was the rest of my year taken care of. I shook his hand again and left, thankful I wasn't going home to organize my funeral.

7

Survival kit

Chemotherapy, what would it do to me? Would I have a bad reaction? Light up like I had a bit part in the Simpsons? The bleak gates of Belvoir Park Hospital did nothing to offer me reassurance. Belvoir was an old Victorian sanatorium, the very mention of which struck fear into many. It hadn't changed much since the turn of the century. In its favour, it was set in rolling parkland, but that did little to distract your attention from the red brick, prison-type buildings with their high windows. It had a haunted feeling, like it was a place full of spirits... perhaps those not lucky enough to go back out the tall gates.

The lump in my breast was gone but the lump in my throat which arrived with the bad news on 16th March grew tenfold. I felt as if I was suffocating. Overwhelmed by it all, I just wanted to run and keep running, to anywhere but here. But I had to go in and face it. A few weeks earlier, the consultant had explained that there was a 30% chance of my cancer returning. Now I'm not a betting person, but I didn't rate my odds. So where else could I go, I had no choice.

Surprisingly, Belvoir was warm and almost homely. No one looked ill or dying. Badly fitted wigs were the only telltale signs of who were the patients. Many sat around heartily tucking into sandwiches and soup provided from a little kitchen in the corner – a sight which reminded my stomach that I hadn't really eaten since March. My clothes size had dropped to a size eight or six and my frame was looking quite small in my jeans and pink top, but that aside, no one would have guessed that I was a patient either. Strangely, primary cancer doesn't make you look ill, it's the treatments that do that. But secondary or terminal, well, you're more easily spotted with those ones.

My guts were now churning, though I'm not sure if it was from nerves or from the smell of the chicken soup. However, the nurse delegated to administer my treatment was excellent, her confidence and professionalism allayed all my fears. She explained all the drugs, their side effects and the side effects of the side effects. In front of me sat a kidney dish full of horse-sized syringes, all with my name on them: drugs to kill the cancer cells. The 'big guns' for someone who could fall asleep on two paracetamol!

The nurse was gowned from head to foot, goggled and gloved – a splash was to be avoided at all costs – but for the patient there was to be no such protection. The drugs careered through my arterial system at speed. They were a colourful array of poisons, especially the sarsaparilla one with its sweet pink appearance, fooling me into a false sense of childlike comfort. It would kill all my hair before a fortnight was up. As each syringe was injected into my veins I wondered how they found the cancer cells. But that was a daft thought. The drugs weren't that smart. They didn't look for a needle in a haystack, they just demolished the haystack.

A half hour later I felt a bit queasy when I stood up but I

think that was more fear than drug induced. I walked out of the waiting room, and through the double doors. I had made it. My first chemo was in the bag and I was still standing. I filled my lungs with the fresh, warm, May air and said a quiet, little prayer.

I felt good. I went shopping with Patrick, bought groceries, and went home and made the tea for the kids coming in from school. My parents called with an anxious look on their faces but that soon dissolved when they saw me. Yes, all our fears were unfounded... or were they?

7 pm and whack! A juggernaut hit me when I wasn't looking. My head opened, my stomach churned, my bones ached and I felt violently ill within minutes. I just had the energy to crawl up to bed, pull the duvet over my head and lie there motionless till the middle of the next day. The steroids kept me from sinking in those first few days, but it was no picnic in the park. My body felt as if it was under a huge, internal attack and all I could do was helplessly watch from the sidelines.

Three very long days later, I came back. 'Normality' resumed. If a three day, aggressive, flu-like illness was the worst it would do to me, I thought I would be able to cope. But I needed a plan. I had to start buying more fast foods for the bad days and I needed something to keep me occupied in my tired days.

Knitting! I'm not a great knitter but I'd tried over the years to produce the traditional matching jumpers and cardigans for the girls. Pom-poms for Christmas and bunnies for Easter. They never looked like bunny rabbits but little ones would accept that if their mum said they were bunny rabbits, then they were bunny rabbits. I was happier with a sewing machine in front of me as I could buy a piece of material in the morning and have it on the girls that evening, but it took me a month to finish a little jumper. Months were what I now had to fill.

So, courtesy of Yellow Pages, Patrick and I drove to a wool shop up the Hannahstown Hill. Wool filled the shop from ceiling to floor, it was like walking into a beautiful rainbow. Oh, this was going to be fun. Pattern books challenged me with pictures of arans and mind-blowing designs, but I knew my limitations – plain without too much structure and, if possible, thick wool and fat needles, quantity over quality every time. Armed with enough wool to knit Ireland a little coat, I went to the lady who sat knitting behind the counter.

'You have picked healing colours,' she said.

I took a step back. She couldn't have told I was ill as the chemo hadn't taken its toll yet, but here she was telling me I'd picked healing colours. I felt brave enough then to tell her I was getting cancer treatment and thank her for her comment. At that she slipped a little prayer into my parcel, and I headed home eager to knit my healing jumper. Had I been sent another angel to help me along my journey – my wool angel? The strange thing was that the next time I went to buy more wool, the unit was empty. My shop and my angel had gone.

I finished my jumper, a multi-coloured disaster everyone jokingly begged me not to wear. But when I had bad moments I would wrap myself in it and hope my angels would protect me. Everyone got a disaster that year. The youngsters first, then I worked my way up through the ranks. If you were one of the lucky ones, you got away with a woollen scarf that you could lose in a cloakroom somewhere. But the clack of those needles kept me going, and finishing each item was a challenge as the chemo repeatedly kicked in over the next few months. They weren't just jumpers to me, they were my survival kit.

8

Cancer in the park

Ten days after chemotherapy, my bloods were taken to assess the infection risk. The period from days ten to fourteen is when the body is most susceptible, as the chemo is attacking all the red and white blood cells. Mine were reacting too well. I had a neutrophil count of .0004 – hardly a white cell left to fight any bug or bacteria! So I was packed off home with double antibiotics and basically told not to breathe for four days.

That didn't work. I had just finished setting up Patrick's birthday tea at 6 pm, called everyone in, nicked a pink marshmallow from the cake and BANG! The juggernaut was back. But this time it had brought the entire fleet. I thought I was going to pass out. Shivering, sweating, hot and cold, the marshmallow stuck in my throat waiting to be thrown up. I left them to it and climbed into bed. But one dressing gown and two quilts on that warm, May evening did nothing to heat me up. My head was exploding, I needed dark, I needed quiet, I needed the world to stop. By 9 o'clock I still couldn't shake it off. I was scaring myself, so I phoned Fred, my GP, my boss, my friend, who came within half an hour. One look, one phone call, and I was admitted to Belvoir Park.

This time I didn't notice the big gates or the parkland, I just wanted to crawl into a bed and die. Maybe that night I nearly got my wish. My temperature wouldn't break, I was soaking in sweat, my head was opening, my body lay paralysed on the mattress, and the room wouldn't stop spinning. Then everything went strangely calm and silent and little, keyhole shaped people started walking through the walls. I felt them filling the room. Had they come for me? If so, I had no strength to stop them. Thankfully, a big night nurse held my wrist and counted my weak pulse every fifteen minutes, and didn't let go.

Daylight came. I knew I'd made it through. But I felt very ill. Sore body, sore head, sore mouth, even my skin was sore, and to top it all, the pillow was covered in my hair. I was very frightened that day. My tears, salty from dehydration, burned as they trickled over my face. I wanted someone to make this all stop but no one could. I'd been to hell and back, but I'd survived. Neutropenic Sepsis kills 40% of its victims, the consultant informed me. I wondered how close I'd come to being a statistic.

I spent the rest of the week in bed, and got a little stronger. The children weren't allowed to visit due to the risk of further infection but by Saturday the Ward Sister said I could go home and see them for a few hours. So, venflon in hand and feeling very weak and wobbly, I headed home for hugs and cuddles. But within the hour I found myself cooking lunch and putting in a wash. Now, I'm not sure that was meant to happen. But pampering was not on my menu. It made me wonder just how ill I needed to be before the voice inside me would speak out.

Maybe if I had curled up in a corner and wallowed in misery

someone might have noticed. Not my style, but it didn't stop me yearning for someone to take this weight from me. Patrick supported me through my hospital visits and treatments but he wouldn't mention my illness. A colleague of his had lost his wife to breast cancer a short time earlier. The same could now happen to his wife. He wouldn't ask me questions. He couldn't deal with the answers.

I protected the children, who were too young to really understand what was happening. I was a normal mummy, bald but normal. I saw to the cooking, cleaning, and baking. I organized eighteenth birthdays, Eleven Plus celebrations, new school uniforms for big school, and sixth year formals. It was difficult trying to finish Emma's dress but I got there. She was so beautiful on the night. I had a pre-formal party for her, the same as for Sam the year before. It took place only three days after my sixth chemo, so I was very glad to watch the tail lights of the limo leave the driveway. But the important thing for me was that it gave us another special memory. Normality was good. I needed my children to know normal, I needed my children to remember me as normal.

My parents were devastated by my diagnosis and went into denial, in the hope that if they didn't talk about it, it might disappear. I was their little girl and I had cancer. Cancer killed. Their daughter could die. Why would any mum or dad want to face that? It was the same with my lovely, fairy-godmother aunts. They also took refuge in, 'this can't be happening'. An aunt of theirs, my great-aunt Frances, had died from breast cancer. So denial became their best form of defence.

My big sis was there for me from day one, with her large

boobs nearly drowning me in a big hug; warm and safe where, for a few seconds, my cancer fears disappeared. We'd had many ups and downs over the years, as all sisters do, but just as when we were very small and had to jump on the back of the open bus home from school, she held my hand tight so I wouldn't fall off. She never let go then and I knew she wouldn't let go now.

Brothers were great, walking the walk on the sidelines, cheering me on to the next, poisonous milestone. One found it difficult to cross the starting line, but it wasn't because he didn't care, it was because he did, so he stayed away.

Best friends, Katy and Claire, stood shoulder to shoulder with me every day. Others only braved calling on the good days; and then there were those who must have forgotten where I lived or lost my number. Saying something is better than saying nothing; or saying nothing but just being there. Sadly I watched as some walked in the opposite direction to avoid me. Outside I may have changed, but inside I was still me, that little person, who wanted to giggle, dance and have fun. Laughter was my medicine, people my sunshine. I needed both to make the dark days brighter.

*

Treatments came and went along with the summer and with it any hint of energy I used to possess. I was slowing down. Climbing stairs was difficult, and I could only clean the Monster in spurts. Day to day tasks were taking forever. I felt like Alice in Wonderland with everything growing huge around me. The simple task of washing the kitchen floor or changing the beds rendered me useless for at least an hour. For the second half of my chemo, treatment cycles five to eight, I received Taxane. My consultant recommended me for this new research drug due to the aggressive nature of my cancer. But the treatment was wrecking me. I was now grey and bald, with burnt feet, aching bones and unbelievable fatigue. Not a pretty sight.

Unlike the first four, which hit hard but disappeared after three days, this chemo crept slowly through my body like poisonous ivy wrapping itself around me until I felt completely suffocated. I'd had enough. I was too tired to care. I didn't want any more. While waiting for chemo number seven, I went outside and sat on the kerb wondering if I should just lie down on the road and end it all. But then I felt a wee shoulder to my left. It was my small son. I looked at his little, worried face staring at his sick mummy and from somewhere I gathered the strength to stand up, take his hand in mine, smile at him, and go back inside. I had to keep going for him and my other five, little pearls. I needed to fight this for them. But as I walked back through those double doors I thought about the patients who didn't have loved ones to lift them to their feet. What stopped them from lying in front of a car and ending it all? Maybe faith? The final weapon for my journey.

I would say I have a strong faith. A private faith, not an altar hugging type. Lighting a candle in an empty church does it for me. Since I was fifteen I had a strong devotion to Our Lady. My O Levels, my nurse finals, my love life and my children – yes, she knew it all. I didn't always get what I prayed for, but I usually got what I needed. But this was a big request, maybe even too big for her. I wasn't asking not to die, I was just asking to live long enough to see my little gang blossom. Leaving them was not on the cards. I had so much still to tell them, to teach them, I needed to hold them, to love them. I couldn't do that from another world.

Death doesn't frighten me; it's just another road on life's great journey. It will hopefully take me to the place where I will find my lovely grandpop again, and all the angels who have guided me through life. From my guardian angel, that I left a little bit of my seat for in primary one, to the ones today that lift me to my feet when my own wings are forgetting how to fly. My faith was my ace card.

The chemo had totally changed my physical appearance. My weight had ballooned. From being seven stone ten, I had become a nine stone ten, drug-induced puffball, with a potato head, no hair, no eyebrows and worst of all, no eyelashes. My eyes had gone. You can tell a lot about what people are thinking from their eyes – the windows to the soul. I looked into mine, they were dead. No dancing, no fire, no life. Chemo had robbed me of my soul. My eyes had been replaced by two black, lifeless, hollow sockets. My face had become a pallid death mask. Yes, the chemo was working.

Baldness was never a big problem. Once my hair started falling out, Patrick shaved my head and I embraced the Sinead O'Connor look. It was quite freeing not to worry about bad hair days. I travelled to Newry to a wig shop, bought one very similar to my own hairstyle and colour, then left it in its box under the bed. Instead, I bought sarongs in pastel shades, cut them in half and spent the next few months accessorizing them with earrings, bangles and beads. Bows at the back, bows at the side, even plaited bows; I was having a creative ball. Luckily, 'boho' was in that year, or I would have been mistaken for mystic Meg's younger sister. Layers of gypsy skirts and dresses retained the last remnants of my femininity. Never buying into the baseball cap brigade, I hadn't much left to work on, but trying to at least look pretty on the outside made me feel loads better inside.

I experimented with styles. Walking in the anti Iraq War protest with my bald head and parka, I was sure someone was going to ask me if I lived in a tree somewhere to save a forest, or to strap myself to a nuclear fence. Little did they know I was more toxic than any nuclear bomb. I had my lesbian look for the practical day-to-day chores, for the flowing gypsy dress didn't lend itself to cleaning windows or washing dishes. Vest top, combats, and boots may have been more National Front than gay, but I think I got it right when a gay friend said she could fancy me, if I wasn't straight. But sometimes I had a dressing gown look... when I couldn't dig deep enough to put on a happy face. Thankfully, those days were in the minority.

My baldness was something the kids took in their stride, but I did try to cover up when people called, as I sensed their discomfort. My brothers and sister had no problem with it, but my parents and aunts preferred not to see it. It was a raw, too raw reminder to them that I had cancer, and that was more than they could take. My aunts did chuckle though, when one day they brought me new mascara – what I was going to put it on, no one was sure!

Sam and I had a fun day with false eyelashes. We hit the Mac counter in the hope someone with a bit of know-how could give me my face back. Armed with an expensive bag of goodies, we headed home to experiment. One hour later, I resembled a brothel Madame, certainly not helped by the two crawling, spider lashes we stuck to the tips of my eyelids. We laughed so much one made its escape, never to be found again. It was back to the blank canvas.

9

Painting the Forth Bridge

November's dark days arrived, and with them my final chemo. It had been a long seven months since those first, horse-sized syringes on that sunny, warm, May day. Visits to Belvoir Park were now very much routine as I settled myself into the soft armchair beside Patrick, with a book for my final hour of poison.

I had become a regular, I knew all the nurses' names, I knew the programme, I knew what to expect and I could now even tolerate the strange smelling, chicken soup. I had earned my badge. Well, almost. Chemo decided to leave my body the same way it had entered, with a good dose of septicaemia, ten days after the poison-filled drip had been removed. Though not as aggressive as my first dose, I was still admitted until my bloods improved, and rather than delay my radiotherapy, I was started on it while still an in-patient.

The radiotherapy part of the journey was a lot easier, as I was the map. My breasts were tattooed and gridded with blue ink. Similar to the Battleships game my brothers used to play, the radiation searched the grid, found the tattoos, and fired. The cancerous enemy was to be blown up, scattering radioactive debris all around the surrounding tissue. I had to have a heart echo as I would be getting zapped over my heart, and no one could safely say my ticker wouldn't be damaged. There is always a price to pay.

Following my discharge the family took turns to bring me to the remaining twenty sessions. This was lovely, as it gave me time with my dad and my brothers. I knew it was tough on my dad. Belvoir to him was a place people went into and didn't come out of, and here he was driving his daughter in like a lamb to the slaughter. Dads think they should be able to fix everything, but even my dad couldn't handle this one. So just like when I was that little four year old schoolgirl and he was handing me over to the nuns, he delivered me to the radiotherapy door. But this time I didn't cry or plead with him to take me home. I wanted to, but I didn't.

Life was now on the turn, radiotherapy was a stroll after chemo. As I lived locally, I was given the early morning appointments, leaving the later appointments for those who had to travel further. Some who found travel impossible were admitted Monday to Friday, while their relations stayed in chalets in the park grounds.

Arriving for my 9 am appointment, I would be taken into the X-ray room, with its heavily fortified, iron-lined walls, positioned on a trolley and left there for five minutes, while the radiation beamed into my left breast and under my left arm. It was no worse than a standard X-ray. The radiographers returned to the room when it was safe, unstrapped me and I returned to the waiting room. I was home in time for breakfast – or, on the week my dad took me, we shared pots and pots of hot coffee and warm buttered scones in our local cafe.

By now I had bum-fluff hair and was feeling well enough to enjoy my time off. Every afternoon I'd take a short walk around the Belfast Castle grounds before the kids came in from school. Then, rather than go to bed for a nap, I'd doze in the chair watching Ready Steady Cook. Impressed by these televised, culinary delights, I filled my kitchen with gadgets, and home-made soups and freshly baked breads became the order of the day. I was sewing, knitting and painting around the house. Normality was resuming in time for Christmas, just three days after my treatment ended.

I'd made it to the finish line! I was determined to make Christmas 2002 a celebration of living. The tree was the biggest I could find. The presents were the best I could buy and most importantly, I planned to spend every moment with my family and friends. I had made it to the end of a horrible year and from here on each day would be special. I no longer looked on my future as a foregone conclusion. It had to be earned. Christmas, birthdays, holidays – all had to be cherished. That way, if it all ended, I would have no regrets. Sadly though, some things never change. I made the Christmas dinner on my tod.

*

In January, I returned to work, bald and tired. Staying off wasn't an option. The Monster's bills had to be paid, cancer or no cancer. On reflection, it was a crazy thing to do, but it seemed right at the time. I was given paperwork duties in the office for a few weeks. At home I was back on top of everything, and I even joined the gym. Who was I kidding? I was trying to fool everyone, including myself, that I had beaten this. I fell right back into my old ways, not delegating at home or work. I was soon back in free fall.

The night of my daughter Sam's twenty-first birthday, I came over very strange. It felt like the septicaemia. I couldn't wait to get home and crawl into bed. I blamed work as it had been very busy. I had been arranging weight management talks for the patients on top of my normal surgeries, so I thought I was just a bit burnt out from the pressure. But the symptoms got worse, my head was opening, my bones ached and no amount of paracetamol could take away the throbbing in my brain. Luckily I was due for my check-up at the cancer centre in two weeks, so I bided my time.

At the check-up, the consultant took one look at me and organized a bone and brain scan. The next morning, at around 9 am, I was with a patient when my mobile rang. It was the consultant saying she had organized an emergency brain scan for 11 am and I was to come straight over and not to drive... this sounded serious. Did she think I had something growing in my brain? I cleared the next few patients who were waiting, as somehow it bought me time to process the phone call. A little voice inside me was saying, 'Tidy everything up, just in case'.

Patients were wishing me a Happy Easter as I left. It was Holy Thursday again!

My prayer in the brain scanner that day was, please let it be in my bones if it's to be anywhere. I didn't want to not recognise my children and I didn't want their last memory of me to be of a 'lala' mummy. Bone pain I thought I could cope with.

My prayer was answered more fully than I had hoped.

Rather than leave me to sweat it out over yet another Easter, the consultant checked the results there and then. Clear scans! It was a post-chemo viral fatigue. Her advice was to slow down. I had to learn to let go, and take time out.

But how? By now my six children were growing fast, and like any teenagers, their mess was spreading like wildfire throughout the house. Large rooms to give them space turned into a nightmare. It was like painting the Forth Bridge. Get to the end and it was time to start back at the beginning. The house never emptied. Friends slept over, boyfriends filled the dinner table. Some days I could be feeding twelve or eighteen. My kitchen was always full of comings and goings. I loved having so much life around me, but it did take its toll. How was I going to take time out from all this? I was trying to cram as many memories as possible into my life. So I didn't really manage to cut down, but the cancer didn't come back either. At the time that seemed like success. But looking back, '03 and '04 were really years of limbo.

2005 arrived with a bang. A heavy ceiling fell in the study, causing months of devastation, builders' mess, disagreements with insurance companies and a damaged computer. All too reminiscent of 2002. Would the Monster ever give us a break? It was back to arranging building around home life. I used the skills honed from the first time and juggled the balls in the air. But Groundhog Day was complete when I discovered another lump in the other breast. The balls all fell through the floor.

2002: breast cancer. 2004: brain scan and bone scan. And now, 2005: breast lump again. I poked and prodded this new lump in the shower, checking if it was mobile, but it didn't want to go anywhere. It was quite close to the nipple so that in itself proved more difficult to examine.

But I wasn't going to panic. I was holding onto the theory that 90% were benign, but I needed a second opinion. I phoned Claire, but she was away at a conference, so I put it out of my head and waited. Three days wouldn't be very long. But three days turned into three weeks when Claire's mum passed away. Her beloved mum, who had fought breast cancer one year ahead of me, died suddenly, leaving Claire and her entire family reeling. She was only in her early sixties. This was no time for my lumps or bumps. I spent the next fortnight trying to give her the strength she had given to me three years before.

Each night I felt the lump and a cold shudder went through my body, remembering how the painter had told me that his mum died of breast cancer when he was only fifteen... the age of my youngest son. The signs were everywhere. I couldn't ignore it any longer. I spoke to Claire, and in the midst of her grief, she referred me for another scan.

A benign cyst!

I should have felt relief, but this time good news didn't help me bounce back. The waves were just getting too big to jump. At home and at work, I had fallen back into bad habits. I wasn't delegating or asking for help. The new NHS contract recently introduced into all GP surgeries had upped the stakes. If the new contract points weren't reached, salaries or even jobs could be in jeopardy. The career I had loved from the age of seventeen was altering significantly. It wasn't healthcare as I knew it. It was now more like a business. The intention behind the initiative was to be more pro-active rather than reactive to chronic conditions. The theory was good, but in practice it created a stressful increase in all our workloads. The contract was weighted towards health promotion, a role I was heavily involved in. I was falling into a dark hole and I couldn't see any hand pulling me out. If anything I felt the hands were pushing me deeper.

Claire came to my rescue. She organized time off work. She offered me anti-depressants, but I thought I would fight this myself, so they were thrown into the back of a drawer, just in case. My friend Katy went on the attack on the home front. She was always very good at telling it as it was. Katy would take no prisoners, regardless of who she offended. My other half was reeling, but changes were needed. Big changes on the outside, but I also needed to change within.

For three years I had I got up and got on with life with a bravado that even surprised me at times. But inside I was scared, very scared. I was also very sad that life at home hadn't changed. Emotionally, I was feeling isolated. Physically, my immune system was battered. Mentally, I was drained. I was falling to bits. The pieces were so small that no one around me noticed it happening. Life in the Monster continued. To the outside world it was idyllic. Beautiful family, beautiful home, picture perfect marriage. We were an artwork, the envy of many. But like any old masterpiece, begin to look closely and you will see hundreds, thousands, of hairline cracks and flaws.

10

Turning point

2006 was nearly upon us. I threw my heart into the Christmas festivities, putting my feelings into the drawer along with the anti-depressants, to be dealt with another day. But a present that year was to change my feelings and possibly my life forever. Sam bought me Gloria Hunniford's book, Next to You, about her daughter, Caron Keating's journey and ultimate death from breast cancer. I couldn't set it down. I devoured every page, reading late into the night. Her courage and determination to beat this hateful disease was immense. Watching her grow spiritually was like watching spring coming after a long, harsh winter. I cried many tears, but not for Caron. I think they were for me. This book was to become my Bible. When I felt low I would lift it, read a section and be inspired.

But a book can't change the world around you. It had to start with me.

Life muddled along into another new year. It was now almost four years since my cancer. It was starting to become a faded memory, just twelve months away from the big five-year watershed. I don't know what it is about the five-year marker. The medical world groups you statistically into five and ten year survivors. I was very close to earning my first badge. Yet it felt like a hollow victory. My self-made, doormat existence was becoming more and more impossible.

It was Mother's Day, early March 2006. Half way through peeling the carrots for dinner I dropped the knife into the sink, lifted my coat and car keys and blindly drove off down the road. It probably took a while before anyone even noticed that I'd gone as the Sunday football was on telly, and the girls were nursing hangovers from their Saturday night out. Hunger may have been the first inkling that their mother had done a runner. Where was I running to? I don't even remember driving the car, but with tears streaming down my face, I somehow ended up on Waterfoot beach. A beach from my childhood. The beach where I'd learnt to swim. The beach where I'd fished using little nets bought in the one, local shop. The beach where I felt safe.

I was alone. It was getting dark now and quite wet. Everyone had gone home for their Mother's Day treats. My clothes were now soaked through, my straggly, curly hair lashing the sides of my face, but I didn't care. I just kept standing there. I had no idea how much time had passed but the darkness was settling on the water, and all around warm lights were inviting people into the cosy indoors. I stood looking out over that cold sea. Was this a breakdown? Or was this me being sensible for the first time ever? I talked through my tears to my grandpop, begging him not to leave me. I'd never felt this vulnerable and lost before and I was frightened what I might do. At that moment I looked down and at my feet was the most beautiful feather. I wasn't alone!

My mobile ringing startled me back to reality. It was a very distressed Sam wondering where I'd gone. Behind her, I could hear contrite voices in the background and at that moment I knew I had to go home. I had fought cancer for them. I wasn't going to walk away now from my most precious pearls, but I needed a coping strategy. I had made a rod for my own back. Now I had to break it.

11

Meditation in a marshmallow bed

In her story, Caron Keating had sought spiritual solace. Through this path she was able to process her thoughts and fears. I couldn't afford to up sticks and move to Australia as she had done but I could afford to visit my sister for a reiki treatment.

Reiki is a form of alternative healing and meditation through the use of the body chakras and energy sources. A reiki master would hold her or his hands over you, and you may feel yourself transported to wonderful, healing places. Sometimes your experiences can be painful, but most times they are moving and beautiful. That has certainly been my experience.

My first experience though, was not a good one. In 2003 my sister bought me a gift of a reiki treatment for my birthday with another reiki master. This came only three weeks after I had finished my treatment and, looking back, I think it was too soon. I entered her dark, mysterious room where scents enveloped me. During the first part of her reiki, I felt that I was in a cosy, warm cocoon, a happy, safe place where I could heal myself. This was lovely. I felt the light and heat of the cocoon all around me. It was almost womb-like in its sensation.

I felt that I was floating in a bubble, and nothing could

penetrate or damage its walls. Rainbow colours danced round my head, and I felt a deep, calm serenity. But then, near the end, the visualisation took me to a field or garden surrounded by fencing while Patrick and the kids stood up on the hill. This part was scary as I felt that it was my grave, and that the family were on the hill without me. I was too raw and maybe not ready for this treatment, as death and the fear of leaving my children behind were probably uppermost in my mind.

It was with some hesitation that I lay down for my second reiki. But this time, the master was my sister. She wouldn't take me to dark places, so I lay down on her couch and embarked on the first of what would be many, beautiful journeys. Trusting her, I let myself be transported to wondrous places. My mind was free to release all its thoughts safely within this serene world. My body seemed so light I felt I soared through the air, as if carried on wings. I swooped down over fields of yellow flowers and up again. I was flying! I cannot explain in words the exhilaration I was feeling. If you take every beautiful emotion and thought in the world, and roll them all up together, that is how this moment felt.

I then flew towards a brightly coloured kite that was blowing in the wind in front of me and made my way down its string to its little owners. There in front of me stood my children, not as they are today, but as they were ten or more years ago. I saw their happy, laughing faces as they had fun on a sunny day. I could feel them, touch them, smell them.

Then I soared upward again until I came to a garden with a pond. In the garden a barbecue was cooking, and little ones were running about. I could see my children all grown up with their own little ones. Were they my grandchildren, these small little curly-headed people? Then Michael, my eldest drove up in a red sports car.

Flying upward again, leaving this beautiful sight behind, I found myself in Africa. Dusty soil, strong heat on my face, and in my arms a small, black baby. Her small frame was so light to hold, while her new-baby smell filled my nostrils. Around me ran other little children and they seemed to know who I was. The lands around were rural with an odd hut built here and there. Food was cooking on fires, and a gathering was getting under way in a church or school-type, open building opposite. I felt that I was a part of the occasion, not someone looking in on it.

Then I was in a raft going up a river like the Amazon. I could feel the damp heat on my face and hair. The smell of dense foliage rose on either side, while the water was still and murky. Finally, I was being collected from these travels by my children. It was Christmas, with the house decorated and inviting, the big tree glistening in the corner, the food cooking in the oven. I sat down in the middle of my gang, and at that moment my son Michael walked through the door with his new baby.

What did all this mean? Had I been given a glimpse of my past, present and future? When I sat up after this phenomenal experience, I felt for the first time that I had a future. A future that was beautiful, peaceful and calm. I so wanted that future. My grey pallor gave way to rosy cheeks and sparkling eyes. This was the turning point in my healing process. I felt exhausted yet exhilarated. I couldn't wait for my next one. Reiki was to become my life-line in the year ahead.

My sister said an angel, Jophiel, came into her head during
the session. Who was he? I needed to find out more. I did some
research and discovered that he is the angel who can dispel
SAD (Seasonal Affective Disorder); he comes in his gold and
yellow robes to put light back into your life. The archangel of
awakening, wisdom, illumination and joy, he restores happiness.
People could call upon him when they felt the sunshine had gone
out of their lives. He could also be called upon if you wished
to awaken a deeper understanding of yourself, or if you were
searching for answers to questions in your life. That sounded
about right for me.

But I needed more information so I headed to the angel
shop on Botanic Avenue with Sam. Right on the corner of the
street, it was a shop crammed with alternative therapies, angel
books, CDs and crystals. The smell of incense wafting through
the door invited the most cynical of passers-by to step in and
browse. It was quite busy today, lots of hustle and bustle, so Sam
and I made our way to the crystals to find a suitable stone. I was
so engrossed in my task that I failed to see a woman approach
me:

'Why are you not healing yourself?' she asked.

I was completely dumbfounded. Then she said, 'Do you
know anything about healing?'

So I told her I was a nurse to which she replied, 'You give all
your healing away.'

Then she waved her hand over my left breast and arm, and
told me I had no immune system, and that if I didn't start
to heal myself I would get ill again. How did this complete
stranger know so much about me? And why was she giving me

this prophecy of doom? Meanwhile to my right, Sam's mouth was gaping wider with every sentence she uttered. What was I to do with this information? I couldn't process any of what she had said. I had to heal myself? How?

I sheepishly asked her what I needed to do, and she said I needed to get rid of all the emotional baggage that had been weighing me down since early childhood. She said that an event at that time had been the trigger factor. But what?

I rushed home eagerly to relay this to my sister. She said that that particular woman was a top psychic, but she didn't practise anymore. Well, she had just practised on me, that was for sure! Why had she picked me out of her full shop? Had I been taken there to be given that message? Whatever the reason, it stuck with me. Maybe she was right.

I am a strong believer that everything happens for a reason; signs are everywhere, we only need to open our eyes to see them. Something or someone had made me go to her shop that day to receive her message, but now what? Should I ask my parents what happened when I was little, or should I try to work it out myself as I peeled back the layers with each reiki?

Patrick disagreed with reiki, saying it was messing with my head. He thought his wife was going through a breakdown, a midlife post-cancer crisis. But actually, his wife had never felt more in control of her life. I was about to take back the control I had lost many years ago. I was in charge of healing myself. I had done the medicine, now was the time for alternative healing. I could no longer hope that Patrick would understand this spiritual path I needed to embark on, nor could I expect him to walk it with me. At this, I felt very sad.

*

My second reiki was very different to the first. I was the only person in it. Again, I felt transported. All around me were miles and miles of warm, golden beach. I lay reading book after book and then as the sun was setting, I strolled barefoot along the water's edge. This was a very new experience as I had never been one for having quiet time. Only the gentle lapping of the waves disturbed the silence. As I sat down to watch night falling, I felt the presence of a most beautiful angel by my left arm. She was dressed in white and gold, soft, flowing layers, with blonde, silvery hair cascading down her back. Gently she took my hand and guided me to a little, white cottage at the edge of the beach, standing guard on the door while I slept in a big, marshmallow bed with a white feather on the pillow. I sank into a deep sleep that I had never felt the likes of before.

My third reiki was possibly my favourite, as I was walking along skipping and jumping beside my grandpop in my favourite white and red dress, my small three year old hand safe in his. He was not going to let go till he had to. I got the feeling he was trying to tell me he would always be there for me. We walked for miles through a forest with the sunlight glinting between the tall trees. As we came near the edge of the dense woodland I could see a clearing in front of us and in it stood Patrick. When I looked down my little red and white dress had gone and so had my grandpop. I was now a fully-grown woman. But then Patrick disappeared, and I was standing at the top of a mountain being held by a male figure in a warrior costume similar to that of a samurai. He held me in his arms and we flew off to many different worlds.

I didn't always understand the significance of the things I had seen in my reiki but they never hurt me. And I always came round feeling more contented and healed. Reiki was peeling the layers back, taking me into new waters. My fourth session wasn't exactly painful, but it was definitely sad.

I was back on a beach, but this time in winter clothes and my grandpop came and stood beside me. I couldn't move because I had shackles chaining my feet and arms to the ground. The skies were grey and heavy and all around there was a bleakness I'd never seen in any previous reiki. With him were four angels who worked to free the bolts from each shackle. Suddenly I was free. The heavy metal clasps had gone from my wrists and ankles, I could now move. I looked down at myself and my clothes were now light and summery, a sarong and a bikini top, and the cold, winter weather had been replaced by warm sunshine. My grandpop said he couldn't stay, but he would leave Jophiel to take care of me. Then he left with the other angels. They carried my shackles far out to sea and dropped them in the deep ocean. I could feel heavy tears rolling down my cheeks onto my sister's couch.

This reiki made me feel more than ever that things had to change. I appreciated that I was still alive after three years. I had seen four Christmases, four Easters, and four summers. I had watched the cherry blossom bloom in the garden each spring. Every time I saw those delicate, pink, fluffy flowers I thanked God that I'd been given another year. A year to see my children grow into beautiful adults, pass exams, start university and do everything most teenagers do, and most parents take for granted. But for me each year was more precious than the one before. Reaching the five year mark was my goal and I was nearly there. I was lucky. Some of my patients who had been diagnosed with breast cancer at the same time as me were no longer around. Maybe life is a lottery and it depends what queue you are standing in. Who knows? But by this winter all I knew was that scans, scares and lumps were buffeting me, but I was still here jumping the waves.

*

Empowered to change following this latest reiki, I started with the easier shackle.

I was no longer happy at work. Tensions as a result of the new contract were high, moods were low. I had two choices; I could stay or walk. I had got as far as writing my resignation a few months earlier, but a long phone call from Gary, one of the GPs, made me re-think my decision. Walking wasn't really an option as deep down I loved my work and the staff I worked with. I knew this could be sorted if an effort was made. Christmas was only weeks away so this was as good a time as any. Fred and I had always had a good relationship in work, but the demands of the contract had created a tension between us. As my GP, he had walked the walk with me, visiting me in hospital during my three admissions. As a friend, he had eaten his sushi lunch at my house when he visited me on my chemo days. But now as his nurse practitioner, I needed to talk to him in his capacity as one of my employers. So, armed with a poinsettia plant, I drove to his home, bravado deserting me as I stood at his door. What if it goes pear shaped? Maybe I should turn and run. But no, my finger was on the doorbell... too late.

Fred's wife, Jackie, opened the door, closely followed by Fred with a slightly quizzical look on his face. But I think he knew why I was there. In his kitchen one hour ran into two, then three. My eyes frequently filled up, but somehow I kept going. All my anxieties, fears and stresses about work were laid bare, and Fred listened. Then the shackle was dropped in the ocean. He stood up, came over to me, and gave me a big hug. All was going to be OK in work. I just knew it.

The shackles of home life, now that wasn't going to be so easy. But something had to be done. My circumstances were impossible. I thought for everyone, organized for everyone, did for everyone, lived for everyone. I just forgot to live for myself. After Christmas I started sending my mountain of ironing away. Not a monumental change but it was a start. I was delegating for the first time in my life. Yet I still couldn't really make the changes I should have. Those shackles were too long there to remove. So things muddled along, the shackles making a clanging sound, but the bolts never loosening.

Well, not until May 2006. I'd been jumping the waves for four years but this one was to take me down.

12

Grandpop

I had decided to go with the cancer group to Lourdes. This would be the first time since my marriage that I would be away on my own, so I was excited and apprehensive at the prospect. I needed time alone to sort out my head, as it was still all over the place. My final reiki before this trip was grandpop telling me I wasn't listening as he pulled me out, yet again, from under mountains of baggage. He said he was sending a message through my aunt and that I needed to listen. Funny, she gave me the money for Lourdes. Was this his message? Go to Lourdes? Pray, meditate and find myself?

My grandpop had been a big influence on my life. From a very tiny age I loved this short, balding, cuddly, fat gentleman. Short in size, but big in love. My earliest memories were sitting in the back of his Cambridge car with my Big Sis, the leather seats burning my legs as we headed off on exciting, summer journeys. Stopping for ice cream sliders that were too big to hold in one hand; the white, greaseproof paper slippery from the melting cream as it dripped its way onto our new frocks. My grandmother's tuts in the front seat that he should have bought smaller ones fell on deaf ears. Bangor, Bundoran, Portstewart, Dublin – all with a treat at the end. Sometimes very big ones when we would be booked into swanky hotels, or be taken to Fairyhouse to watch the colourful jockeys. Or maybe to the Royal in Bangor where my Big Sis and I played endlessly in the funny lift with its wrought iron doors – much, I'm sure, to the annoyance of staff and patrons alike.

Nothing was too much bother for him where we were concerned. He spoilt us with gifts and clothes from his travels around the world, and every Sunday after mass we got our Sunday sweets from his shop. Except for Lent, of course, when it had to be crisps for six, long weeks. But it was worth it when the Easter baskets appeared. His shop was in the city centre, a Ladies' Hairdressers, Gents' Barbers and a sweet shop. For fifty years he ran it until 1987 when, in his mid-eighties, he retired. Sadly the shop retired with him as no one in the family was interested in the business. The customers were by now the regulars who had stayed with him from their beehive days, but were now settling for blue rinse perms instead. Granted, perms made a fuzzy return in the eighties, but not blue ones!

In the sixties I loved it when my mum would take me in with her when she was having her highlights done. The ladies' room was a poodle parlour of female delights. Pretty ladies would sit reading Woman or Woman's Own with their heads rollered, netted and tucked under oversized, grey, space-age dryers. On their laps, they held large, cream contraptions which they would use to control the heat, and which made a loud click every time they changed it. The remote control of the sixties.

Perm lotions and dyes wafting in the air, I played at tidying up the neat little trays of clips, perm rollers, and brushes. Bored with this I'd go through to the back and watch my grandpop give someone a short back and sides, finished off with a slick of Brylcreem. If my brothers came with us for a haircut they were perched precariously on a wooden plank spanning the arms of the leather, swivel chair. One wrong move or fidget, and they could go flying into the hand basin. I would take the big brush and sweep around all the big people with an air of great importance. Some men came in for a shave and hot towel. I wasn't too impressed with that as I'd watch my dad shave at home, so I'd just disappear into the sweet shop to bother my aunt.

This was probably my favourite of the three places. I'd climb on a stool and serve very patient customers. The big iron till had large, finger-like buttons requiring two fingers, and it would give you a painful nip if your finger got trapped between a pound and a sixpence sign. Adding and subtracting not being my strong point, my aunt thought it better if I weighed out the sweets, taking them from their big, glass jars with a little, silver scoop on a string, then professionally securing the little paper bags. A very important task for a six year old and I took it very seriously, but I never could get that tucked-in, tidy-bag look. They were more a crumpled mess, and my efforts produced many a smile.

My aunt had worked for many years with my grandpop, and knew almost everyone who came through the door, from the folks changing library books across the road, to the bus men from their depot above, to the passing trade getting their cigarettes on their way to work, or a Mars bar for their break. Some were lured in by the shop's ever-changing window display: eggs, chicks and baskets at Easter, net stockings filled with goodies at Christmas.

My favourite thing of all was the tray of homemade fudge. I had usually sickened myself by home time, having hoovered up all the crumbs and broken pieces.

As I got older I didn't call in as much, unless I'd lost my bus fare or dinner money. When I was studying in the library I would call to say a quick hello, but I no longer wanted to stack the rollers in tidy lines and the pretty ladies were all gone by then. By now the shop was growing old along with my grandpop. Old workers and old customers dwindled down to the loyal few, but he still made the daily journey on the 7.15 am bus every weekday morning, except Monday as that was the hairdressers' day off.

When I worked in the Mater I joined him, sleepy-eyed on this journey. He was always at the bus stop, in his camel raincoat and brown hat, hands behind his back. He didn't need to make this trip. He had made his money, he had built my grandmother a beautiful home, but he did it because it was the job he loved doing since he was fourteen.

So he would go in and muddle along at a slower pace, trapped in his time-warp of short back and sides, even though in the eighties the mullet was all the rage. He would shoo me down the bus, telling the driver and anyone else awake enough to listen that I was running the Mater hospital single-handed. Then he would proceed to tell them how I could peel a pot of potatoes back to front with my klutey hand, and cook for an army while baking him a great cake.

I would lean my forehead against the window, cold from the early morning frost, to grab a few more minutes' shut-eye, smiling to myself at how only a grandpop could love you enough to think you were so perfect. These were good journeys; and now that he's not here I wish I'd kept my eyes open just a little bit more. Now I have to pay my own bus fares and live with my imperfections, as he isn't there to tell me how great I am.

We think people will live forever but they can only do that in your heart. His last years were blighted by confusion and mini strokes. Some days he didn't know any of us. From my grandmother to the great grandchildren he adored, none would register with him. He would talk of going down home to see his mummy and then wander out of the house in the direction of where he was born. If I caught sight of him from my kitchen window, I would coax him inside, playing along with his surreal world until he would return to mine. Then I'd walk him home just round the corner. But his time in the real world was getting short.

His world was eighty years ago and that's where he took himself most days until one damp, October day his brain went there but forgot to come back. His power was gone on one side, and he was semi-conscious when the ambulance took him for the last time from the home he designed and built after the War. He didn't need his camel coat or brown hat for this journey. I never heard my grandpop speak again after that day. No more ice cream sliders, no more Pickie Pool, no more a sweet for your hand and one for your pocket, no more grandpop. In the hospital I fixed his hair. The nurse had combed it to the wrong side. She wasn't to know.

It was a very wet, miserable Hallowe'en day when I stood by that muddy hole in the ground, holding my dad's hand tight as we both said our goodbyes to the man we loved. But I don't go to that graveyard to find him anymore. If I want to talk to him I go to his seat on the porch at Number Three. I still feel him there, taking the air in the evenings, getting his forehead burnt by the late, summer sun. And now, reiki and my sister have given me a chance to see him again. Maybe it is only a picture in my sub-conscious but for that hour it is real, he is real. And it was about time I heeded his messages.

13

Oh no! Not again

Lourdes preparations got under way. We were due to go on the Saturday, so I finished work on Wednesday and made Thursday a day of pampering. A quick haircut, then a spray tan using a birthday voucher, then I'd meet Claire and Biddy for lunch. It was such a beautiful, May day I decided to walk the three miles from the salon to the coffee shop. When I arrived looking tangoed and sweaty, the jokes were flying about wet T-shirts and going bra-less. We were in such a kink none of us saw Fred come in, carrying a piece of paper.

I had asked Fred as my GP to check my mammogram before I headed off. I was very casual about it as this was now my fourth. I just really wanted the results out of the way. But this wasn't casual. When I glanced up, all that my eyes could see was the piece of paper in his hand – my results. Claire and Biddy were gabbing away, totally unaware of this slow motion nightmare unfolding. He sat down facing me and said that the test had shown up an abnormality.

Claire stopped talking. I couldn't talk and Biddy's mouth just dropped. I'm not sure who filled up first, but if Fred had done so too, I'd have known the game was up. Wet T-shirts and fake tans seemed a lifetime away now. The grim reaper had again made an uninvited appearance. Claire kicked into action, trying to get a scan before Lourdes while Biddy said all the right things, but really they fell on the ground. An abnormal mammogram. Would this curse never leave me?

Claire had to go back to work, so Biddy took me up the Cavehill where my tears flowed liked a mountain stream. I was tired of being in this position. This was my fourth scare in four years. Had I not done enough? Had the chemo not worked? What had I left to fight a new cancer with? I'd been given extra doses of chemotherapy; I'd been given new research drugs, so what now? I felt lost and hopeless as I stood looking over my Belfast, my city, my world. The road ahead suddenly looked bleak and dark. Maybe I'd seen my final cherry blossoms.

My youngest was now fifteen, the age the decorator had been when he lost his mum. Maybe as a mother this was the cut off point. Maybe they could now survive without me, but how was I to survive without them... I didn't want to leave my beautiful string of pearls.

I didn't want to be a memory or a piece of cold stone in a graveyard. I couldn't hug or hold or kiss them from afar. I couldn't feel their soft hair when they snuggled up beside me or feel the warmth of their hands in mine. My babies that I'd nurtured from their first feed, first tooth, first steps, first day at school, first romance, first broken heart – were there to be no more firsts? I hadn't seen them graduate, get married, have beautiful babies of their own. Had my first reiki only been wishful thinking? Was this it?

I left Biddy to go light a candle at Our Lady's altar, and for the first time in my life I begged her for more. My mind was racing to dark, eerie places. These were crazy, mad thoughts but for the first time in four years they wouldn't go away. I stayed in that empty chapel and prayed for a miracle.

I needed to go home. I needed someone to hug me and hold me till this madness left my brain. So I waited for Patrick to come in and told him what had happened. He gave me a hug, lifted his coat and left. Could he not cope? I stood alone in the huge mausoleum with its emptiness bouncing off the walls. Patrick had run away... but I couldn't. My right breast was attached to this abnormal mammogram result. At that moment, I knew that emotionally I was on my own.

Claire stepped up to the plate and again organized a scan for the next day, so all I had to do was get through this one. My daughter Emma had just finished university and was starting a new job. So Sam, Bunty and I headed into town with her to get her some new clothes. I was playing my part really well until Sam jumped out of the changing room in the most beautiful black dress saying it was a pity she hadn't a funeral to go to.

My pretence crumbled. I had to tell Sam and Bunty the truth. Emma already knew as she had caught me crying in the kitchen earlier, but I'd sworn her to secrecy. So now my girls knew. Sam fell apart. Emma and Bunty stayed strong, saying they would help me through whatever lay ahead. Suddenly my innocent, young girls became grown-up young women.

*

At 9 am the next morning I lay in a dark scanner room. A probe slid gently across my right, gel-covered breast as the radiologist searched for the culprit that had brought me here. Watching the monitor I could see the darkened mass appear on the screen, and then I felt a fine needle pierce my skin and thread its way into the centre of this blackness. A few twists and turns later its contents were spread onto yet another slide and handed to the histopathologist. I was asked to wait on the couch. It's funny, the small talk that can occur when your life is on the tip of a needle. The radiologist said he'd been off the day before and that's why Claire couldn't reach him. He was having his hair cut. I'd spent my day planning my death; he'd spent his having his locks trimmed. How odd life can be. But his hair did look well.

The histopathologist re-appeared requesting a further biopsy. I couldn't figure out if this was a good or bad sign, so I just lay quiet biting my tongue as another needle wriggled its way under my nipple.

Another needle. Another result. That beautiful, fat, little cell – the fat, little word – benign!

I went home and packed to run away to Lourdes! I needed time on my own to figure out where my marriage was going. We had stopped talking about what was important. Instead we talked about mundane, day-to-day stuff, but never about what really mattered. What I couldn't deal with was the distance that was growing with each test. Was that living? Maybe Lourdes would give me some answers. Maybe time apart would help me see things more clearly. Would this be the beginning of the end of our marriage? Everything seemed finely balanced. Maybe we could put things right. But maybe the cracks could not be varnished over.

14

Lourdes

I t was early, but a long queue had formed at the desk. Everyone seemed to know everyone else. I scanned faces but saw no one from the clinic. So I started to chat to the people beside me and within minutes I think I'd been introduced to the entire line. Everyone went out of their way to be friendly. Some, like me, had been cancer patients, others were patients' relatives, and the remainder were carers. There was a camaraderie there that was really hard to beat.

I wasn't sure what to expect when I got to Lourdes. I suppose I had some reservations that it might be filled with devout, praying people. But it wasn't like that at all. Yes, many were devout and many were there for healing – a cure and maybe even a miracle – but any preconceived ideas I had of it being a place of sickness and death were soon dispelled. It was a place full of life and hope. Coffee shops were buzzing and as evening progressed, pubs were spilling onto the streets with laughter and music. The reverence was saved for the grotto.

During the day processions of people from all nationalities converged on the grotto to queue for the baths. This was a very weird experience. Following a long wait, six or eight ladies and I were shepherded into a concentration camp type of building where Gestapo-type large ladies handed out thin wraps. I sat beside Elaine whose brainwave this had been, wondering how to make my escape. She had been many times and had a very strong faith in the power of the baths. At this moment, sitting naked under a fine cloth with complete strangers, I wasn't sure I was getting it.

My turn arrived. Shooting Elaine a look of sheer terror, I was timidly ushered in behind the curtain, where my wrap was replaced with a thin, wet muslin towel to maintain what was left of my dignity. I was told to walk three steps into a stone bath filled with icy cold water while saying a prayer. Once there, women on either side plunged me backwards into the water. The suddenness of their movement and the coldness of the water combined to stop my breath, but within a few seconds it was over and I was once again back out in the changing area.

Going in, I'd found it strange that no one had brought a towel, but then I realised I wasn't wet and my clothes could be put back on without my having to dry myself. Outside, waiting for Elaine, I reflected on how strange I felt, but I also had a lovely, calm, warm feeling. Maybe she had been right after all.

The Cancer Centre group were good to be with. For the first time in four years I didn't have to hide my fears or pretend, as everyone here felt the same as I did. Cancer was a part of their lives, and together Elaine, Mark, Annie and others empowered me to challenge it, accept it, embrace it, live with it. We shared many special moments; the candle-light procession when we walked proudly as one under the Cancer Centre flag; our tearful healing mass when we were all anointed with healing oils. Then there were also the hotel sing-songs and much banter into the small hours of the night.

Slipping away from these like Cinderella at midnight, I would walk through the deserted streets that had been thronged with tens of thousands just a few hours earlier. Mark had advised that if I wanted to find the real Lourdes, I needed to go at night. So, stealing out through the back gate, down the winding path and past the blind man statue, I hurried on until I found the grotto. There were rows and rows of flickering candles, their wax droplets mirroring the tears shed. Behind me, the dark river reflected the depth of the pilgrims' pain and before me, Our Lady's beautiful statue stood, hewn into the rock. No matter where I moved, her eyes followed, easing my pain and the many tears I shed over my life and where it was going. Hours passed before I realised I was cold and tired, and wet from the spring rains. I had found my spiritual place. A magical place, Our Lady's Grotto. Leaving Ireland on the plane a few days earlier, I had said to Mark, a frequent pilgrim, that I was frightened I wouldn't get it. Now, as I knelt on St. Bernadette's Square at 2 am, I knew I had.

The day we left Lourdes, we dedicated two giant candles in the grotto. One was to burn brightly for our group as we made our journey home and the second was to burn in memory of Dr Gerard Lynch, the consultant who had founded this cancer centre pilgrimage some thirty years earlier, only to succumb to the deadly disease himself.

The trip had given me peace, close friendships and hopefully, the strength that I would need to sustain me through the next, very difficult part of my journey.

*

Arriving home from Lourdes I knew what I had to do. Telling Patrick that I was no longer happy in our marriage was horrible. But nothing prepared me for the nightmare that followed. Minutes later, he came in from the garden where I had spoken to him, set his wedding ring on the dinner table, and announced to his captive audience that their mummy no longer wanted to be married to him.

It was the beginning of the end.

Walton Mountain was no more. This wasn't 1980 when we could walk away from each other relatively unharmed. Six other, very important people were now involved. The fight had begun and all I could do was stand in horror and watch from the cooker as my children fell apart because of me. If he did it to get back at me, it worked. I hated myself at that moment and for every moment of the next twelve months of hell.

Staying under one roof in the middle of a war zone for the good of the children is not to be advised. If anything, it did them more harm watching the adults of the house destroy each other. Us hating each other and them hating us for hating each other. But at no time, throughout the vitriol and condemnation, did I swerve from my path. It was not the easier one to choose. Easy would have been to stay, to return to silence in the beautiful masterpiece. Easy would have been to ignore the million tiny flaws spreading deeper with time. No, this was tough. I had needed every ounce of strength to battle through cancer. I needed still more to get through this.

15

Africa

By October, the war had dragged into its fifth month and reached stalemate. We both dug into our trenches in the mausoleum; no retreat in sight, no truce, no treaty. Someone had to do something to create space for us to breathe.

Following a visit to my youngest brother, John, and a long heart to heart with him, he reminded me how, when he was a boy, I'd talked to him of working in Africa. Maybe this was the time to do it. I had another brother, James, working in a township near Pretoria. I would go to him, seek sanctuary, solitude. Patrick called me selfish and maybe I was, but I needed to go. We were cutting deeper wounds in each other than any knife would be capable of. At least knife wounds can heal; words, once spoken, cannot be taken back.

Cupboards filled, fridge and freezer packed to capacity (and if all else failed, there was always the drawer filled with takeaway leaflets!), I was ready to go. I secured my rucksack and checked for the fiftieth time that I had my little red passport. After tears and hugs from the gang and my team of well-wishers (Big Sis, Janet, Katy and Claire), another brother, Martin drove me off. As he did, I looked back at the mausoleum and wondered if Patrick and I would have been on a different path, but for the Monster.

Dublin airport was buzzing. There was time for a quick burger – and also time for any change of heart – before my brother left. But I knew this was right for everyone. It wasn't a truce, just time-out. So I waved him goodbye, and clutching my boarding pass, I nervously headed through the gates to a world I had dreamed of visiting back in 1978.

Beside the red book, safely tucked in a pocket of my shoulder bag, I carried a thin, blue and white, airmail letter addressed to a naive, young student nurse c/o the Nurses' Home, Belfast City Hospital, all those years ago. To a nurse who had been going to go out and save the world, had her parents let her. Her big plan had been to work for a year in Africa after she qualified, the place where she'd sent her copper pennies when she was four. The place where her and her sister sent pounds after running a fête in their back garden and garage for the starving people of Biafra.

A delay of a year or two wouldn't make much difference. So the nineteen year old nurse had slipped the letter stamped from Malawi into the memory box under her bed and waited. Now, twenty-eight years, one marriage, six children, one nurse practitioner degree, and one breast cancer later, she was on her way.

It was strange to have only myself to think about on the journey. I kept feeling I was missing something, like six children. Usually times spent in airports on family holidays were hectic, to say the least. Clusters of passports, a freight load of luggage, food and drink to be consumed by hungry mouths, toileting at regular intervals, making sure males and females weren't taken at the same time so that one parent would be left to watch the luggage.

Now I could walk around duty free without watching out for an entire shelf of expensive perfume to hit the floor. Without the constant fear, every parent's worst nightmare, that one would go missing. Watching six was a mammoth task, worthy of a mention in David Attenborough's Guide to the Species. This habit was so ingrained in my being that I found myself watching other people's kids as I milled from shop to shop. But after a few suspicious looks from mothers, I found a safe corner and tucked myself up with a book.

On my first long haul I learnt a lot of do's and don'ts:

Don't wear big lace-up boots, for that may cause an irate queue behind you at security as you try to get your pudding feet out of them at the flight changeover, having gained half a stone on the previous flight.

Don't take same boots off on second flight as you will have to walk off plane bare-foot when your feet, now weighing a stone, will never go back into your size threes.

Don't pick an in-flight movie where you spend two hours laughing or crying out loud, forgetting you are the only one tuned into it.

Don't drink too much coffee when you are at a window seat as it creates a huge annoyance to your fellow travellers as you clamber over them for the umpteenth time.

Don't leave Dublin dressed for Africa as the plane is quite cold during the night and the ultra thin blanket given in economy does nothing to ward off hypothermia.

But do enjoy every minute!

The plane was quiet now, but I couldn't sleep – too much nervous excitement and possibly too many coffees, so I watched as the tiny symbol of our plane followed the line on the monitor over the vastness that was Africa. I looked out my window into a clear, dark, navy sky, lit up by a million stars. I wondered how the mothers of Darfur below, displaced from their homes, were keeping their babies warm under this cold night air. At that moment I thought of my own six now tucked up in bed and I shed a tear. It would be four, long weeks till I could wrap them in a hug. But maybe I would come back to them a happier mummy. So I blew a small kiss out the window, hopefully in the direction of home, and hoped it would land safely on their cheeks for now.

Fourteen hours later, with my rucksack claimed, I headed to the exit, and there to my delight stood my brother with a bouquet of flowers. In that moment I knew this would be a good journey. One hour in his truck later, we arrived at the township. I had seen many pictures taken by him and others, but nothing prepared me for Atteridgeville.

It was a small, dusty corner of Africa, filled to overflowing with possibly one million people (though no one had ever taken the time to count them). This was the home of many families that had been uprooted from the cities in the days of apartheid and abandoned well out of sight of white South Africa. Homes constructed mainly of tin on poor ground – with no water, no sanitation and no electricity – were the norm for most.

But these people were proud of their little corner, and during my stay I would watch from my bedroom in the hospice as the women swept the orange soil in front of their homes with bunches of long twigs. They would hang whiter-than-white washing out to dry in the heat of the morning sun, having first washed it in basins of water collected from the large green drums located throughout the township. Though not all the properties were of such poor construction. We drove through a small area where people in the new Mandela era were building better homes, many with water, sanitation and electricity. Most had lived in the township for almost fifty years. They didn't feel the need to go back and re-claim their cities. This was their piece of Africa.

After a very bumpy ride, as the roads were basic, James stopped so I could view his hospice on the hill. This would be my working home for four weeks. I wanted to pinch myself – here I was standing in the middle of an African township, my feet on orange soil, my head in the clouds. My dream was now a reality. At the hospice door I was greeted by the entire staff singing a Seuto welcome song. For the first time in what felt like forever I filled up with happy tears. This would be a good place to heal.

The hospice was run by senior nurses who had all come out of retirement to help my brother. Remija, a strong and beautiful African grandmother, was matron. Her ways were old-school which I liked – time spent with patients, not time wasted writing up too many care plans. It was an eighteen-bed unit. Eight male, eight female and two side wards for the dying. Aids was a disease that had blighted this beautiful country, filling its graveyards with headstones inscribed with birth dates from the nineteen seventies, eighties and nineties. It ravaged the young of this community, leaving the very old to look after the very young. Funerals were an all too common event. Burials on a Sunday could be heard throughout the township.

My brother built this hospice so people could die with dignity in a clean bed, cared for in their final days. For too long he had visited the dying on dusty floors, often without a mattress, the heat from the tin walls ensuring their infections couldn't escape. He came up with this plan and, my brother being my brother, he made it happen.

Now I was a part of this team in my white T-shirt and navy, long shorts. October is the start of the summer there, and they were amused that I wore shorts as some had not yet shed their winter layers of wool. Me, I found it very hot. My shifts were rotated week about. One week I worked 7 am to 2 pm and the following week, 2 pm to 7 pm. On the weeks I finished at 2, I would go up to the nearby crèche at St. George's and help out in the nursery. The little ones were fascinated with my pale skin and blond hair, many never having seen a white woman before. The older children would rub my arms to find my dark skin, and they nick-named me 'big hair', trying to plait my blond curls into braids.

It didn't take long to fit into the hospice. I spent the first week shadowing all the six sisters. They taught me so much, not only about the hospice and the treatments for Aids, but also about their township. Patients mainly came from the township, but sometimes they came from much further. One afternoon I tried to admit a young girl, but without success as she only spoke Zulu. We waited for a night staff nurse who acted as interpreter. Many other languages were spoken, but Seuto was the main one, so I embarked on learning very basic greetings such as 'Salang pila'.

The beds never emptied except sadly when someone passed

away due to this horrible disease. Eleven died during my four weeks at the hospice. Some deaths might have been prevented had patients continued to take their ARV Aids medications, but there was still a strong belief in the old witch doctors, and many preferred their traditional medicine, 'Muti', over more modern treatments. By the time these young people found it wasn't working and came for conventional treatment, it was often sadly too late.

*

I know nurses aren't meant to have favourites, but I couldn't help but love Philip. He was a thirty-three year old with full-blown Aids, tuberculosis, and cerebral atrophy, all the side effects of Aids. Every day he would sing me a Seuto song, and we would dance in the garden, him shuffling in my arms due to his neuropathy. All he ever wanted was a Granny Smith apple, so every morning on the way to handover I would slip into the kitchen and pinch one from Seamus, the volunteer chef. Seamus arrived from Leitrim the same time as me, but he had come by way of Boston and this was his last stop before heading home. We immediately developed a great and lasting friendship.

When darkness fell over Africa at 7 pm, the township could be a dangerous place, so from behind a locked fence we made our own fun courtesy of a few bottles of amarula and lots of laughs. We chatted and sorted each other's problems out into the wee small hours of 11 pm, way past African bedtime. This was a world that woke at 5 am and slept at 8pm, except of course at the weekend when, similar to our Irish ways, they knew how to throw a good party. Then, thirty-six hours of drums and singing could be heard from all over the township. Around the hospice very few homes had electricity so we stood in the dark on the veranda and listened as each perfect note was carried mystically through the night sky, bouncing off the moon, tumbling between the stars and returning to earth even sweeter than it left.

Sunday though, was a different style of music. Partying finished, this was time for the Sunday best – tribal costume for the very special occasions – when the community met up to celebrate life through prayer, dance and song. Seamus and I wondered at what they had to be grateful for in this arid corner of the earth. We grew to realise that their happiness was not measured on the outside but on the inside. To have so little, yet feel contentment, is a value many in the western world could do with learning.

Death was not approached with fear, but seen as a going forward into a bright future. Many patients would be heard to say with a smile on their lips, 'today is a good day to die', and they did so very peacefully. The only fear attached to death was providing for the hundreds and sometimes thousands that would come to the funeral feast. Unlike in the West, when only a handful may turn up, here entire villages turn out for this special occasion and having a cow to kill and cook is a must. Providing no cow means providing a poor celebration of the person's life. Two cows and you were well respected. One patient in the hospice constantly worried over having no cow to feast at his funeral.

I also became great friends with the younger staff, who would take us sightseeing when we were off duty. African markets, safari parks, the Cradle of Mankind and of course, Pretoria. There, we were fed gloriously by my brother's French friend, Franc, with the melting chocolate voice. It was a wonderful month. A month when I had space to find myself and re-build me, at the same time doing something that felt worthwhile. The sparkle in my eyes returned, and grew brighter as it neared home time and the prospect of seeing my little gang again. But I also felt sad at leaving my brother and the lovely people who had taken me into their homes and their hearts.

On our last day Seamus and I were both reduced to mush. The nurses made me a beautiful Seuto costume. A female patient made me a pair of red, beaded shoes. Maybe like Dorothy in The Wizard of Oz, they were a sign I was ready to click my heels and head for home. Seamus was given an African crock-pot for cooking. At the farewell barbecue, Philip and I had our last dance, me in my Seuto dress, him in his pyjamas. My lovely Philip died two weeks after I came home. My prayer when I heard was that his angels would always make sure he had a Granny Smith apple and that he could now dance pain-free, 'like no one's watching'.

*

My next visit to the hospice was not to be the happy event of the first.

Five months after I left, robbers broke in and shot my brother. The family felt helpless back in Ireland. My dad and my brother Francis flew over to be at his bedside. It was felt I would be a better help going out to nurse him when he got out of hospital. So I bided my time and waited with my distraught mum and the rest of the family by the phone for any scrap of news about his condition. Together we were strong, so my brothers and sister stayed at my mum's through the worst of it, only going home to change and freshen up.

My turn soon came. I travelled out with Martin, the same brother who had left me to the airport the first time. When we got to Atteridgeville we felt the community's shock and outrage at first hand. The staff were devastated, the township was devastated. The incident made headlines all across the world. The nightly news and daily papers followed James' progress. By and large, this passed me by. For all I saw was my wee brother lying in a hospital bed, looking very ill.

James was moved to recuperate at the Convent of the Little Company of Mary, a tranquil environment where he would find time to heal not only his physical scars, but the invisible ones as well. Most days, he would sleep for short periods. During this time I would take the intercom with me, as he was understandably frightened to be alone, and sit reading by the small pool in the garden. No way had I envisaged being back in Africa so soon. But here I was on that big, fifth anniversary of my cancer sitting on a swing seat alone with my thoughts.

The nuns were lovely, and hovered over him and I like clucking, mother hens. Food kept appearing on pretty, lace-covered trays, not to mention little treats delivered with his mail. He received hundreds of letters and cards wishing him a speedy recovery, brought by an endless stream of well-wishers. Part of my job was to say 'No more,' when I saw him fading, as he relived the horror of his ordeal with each new visitor.

When he began to get his strength back, Martin, Franc and I would venture out with him, but never too far. And when he was ready we took him back to the hospice. I could only imagine how difficult it must have been for him. We kept the visit short and soon returned to the security of the convent. The outside world no longer felt safe for him. Returning to his old life beyond the locked gates would not be easy.

By a remarkable coincidence, a nun, Sister Kathleen, who had lived beside us in Belfast when we were small children and who had loved my brother dearly, had gone on to work for many years in this convent before she died. When, after three weeks, I had to return home, I prayed to her to look after him and Martin until they too could travel back to Ireland.

16

Moving out

Emotionally, my trips to Africa changed nothing. They didn't bring about the change of heart that Patrick may have hoped for, so the uneasy truce ended. On came the big guns, the estate agents and solicitors. No one ever warns you that a marriage breakdown is like being awake in a permanent nightmare. Each day swimming through toffee to get to the other side and every time you think the bank is within touching distance the toffee pulls you under.

It was now an impossible existence. My brother, Francis offered me the use of a dilapidated house round the corner that he was waiting to demolish. I felt there was no alternative but to accept. If I cleaned it up it would do as a stop-gap until the Monster was sold. It had three bedrooms so there was plenty of room for the kids to come and go between both homes.

Sis, Janet, Katy and I rolled the sleeves up and tried desperately to see the plus side to this property. Many gallons of dirty water later, we sat outside and felt quite pleased with the results. We could have done without the gruesome task of removing seven dead blackbirds, including one that had somehow drowned itself in the toilet. It was amazing what a few bunches of flowers could do to take your eye off the fact that the concrete floor was lifting, the heating didn't work and the bath was a yellowy grey. But the house was mine for now. Tomorrow I would move out and move in.

*

I woke eager to jump from hell at least into limbo. But purgatory awaited me that day. If I was to be punished for my actions this was to be the day it would happen.

My two youngest, John and Anthony, along with my friend Katy's lads, spent the morning painting the concrete floors. Michael had gone to a barbecue the previous night shouting cheerio, my 'I love you' getting trapped in the letter-box as he pulled the front door shut. The children had decided that the three lads would move in with me and the two girls would stay with their dad. Sam had already moved into her own place. That day I spent my lunch break buying duvets and food for the old fridge. At 1.55 pm my mobile rang.

Michael had been in an accident. I grabbed my car keys, told the doctors I had to go and drove like a banshee along the motorway giving no consideration to penalty points. He probably has a broken toe, please let him have a broken toe... please, I prayed.

My eyes scoured Casualty. For a few seconds I couldn't find him, like the time I lost him in Dunnes for all of two minutes and it felt like a lifetime. Where was Michael? Just then, a group of important looking doctors stepped back from a trolley. My heart stopped. There was the mad mane of curls. The pale face. The near lifeless body. It was Michael. My baby boy.

At that moment the nurse said she would take me to the visitors' room. Oh my God, please don't take me to that room. I know why you go there, I've taken so many there myself. But I remained still and quiet, only mumbling to her to please let me see him. Just then, when I thought I wasn't going to get through this moment, my lovely brother, Francis came through the door as if sent by an angel.

Together we stood beside Michael. He was holding onto life by a thread. The pain was unbearable. The labour pains that gave him life, the toughest of all six, paled compared to this pain that his life might be taken away only twenty short years later.

Patrick arrived. We were together again. Strangely but clearly together. United in pain, we needed to get through this for our firstborn son, our precious Michael. For five hours he was in surgery while the entire family circle waited in that visitors' room for news. By teatime he was in intensive care on a ventilator, attached to a multitude of machines. But he was alive and that was all that mattered.

Every night when the family left I would stay on to watch Michael through the Intensive Care Unit's glass partition, just as I had watched him through his little, glass cot in the maternity unit. Watching him breathe, willing him to be whole again. I was too scared to sleep for fear of losing one single moment, or of him not knowing I was there and being frightened. So, snuggled up in a chair, I kept vigil over my curly-haired boy. Sometimes, though strictly not allowed, a nurse would slip me in to sit beside him and hold his hand till the dawn broke and he came closer to making it through to another day.

Five gruelling days later, most of the machines were removed and he was taken, battered and weary, to the High Dependency Unit. The wrecked car he had been a backseat passenger in had mangled his body. His spleen had been removed, his lungs collapsed, his heart shifted, yet, if you didn't count the smashed arm, strangely, he hadn't so much as a scratch on his body.

Now that he had made it to the High Dependency Unit, he was considered ill but stable. Good words which meant I could sleep by his bed every night. One very special night I had dozed over with my head on his bed only to be awakened by the gentle feel of his hand on my hair. I lifted my face and at that he drew three, weak fingers down my hair, over my forehead, eyes, nose, ending at my lips in a gentle finger kiss before he fell back to sleep again.

I was complete again. Sadly, as each day saw Michael improve, Patrick's and my relationship fell apart again. I was being accused of having a breakdown, right words but wrong context – I was being broken down, which is quite different. By now I was too weary to fight anymore. When Michael was better I would go as planned. So after he was discharged, for a while I slept on the floor beside Michael's bed as the drugs and no doubt the crash were giving him nightmares. But with each day his physical strength improved and when I thought he was well enough to move to my halfway home I planned our exit.

But it wasn't to be. Michael decided to stay... but I couldn't. Perhaps it was for the best for him to recuperate in the home he knew, and where it was warm and clean. But I felt that for the next two, long years I had lost him. Maybe he thought the accident would make me stay, have a change of heart. But I hope some day he will understand how painful it was to go... that I never abandoned him. Just like his first days at school, when I watched him from a nearby car park to make sure he was safe, now I had to do the same again, watch him from a distance.

17

New home, new start!

The Monster was sale agreed, Patrick had a new home sale agreed, I had to act fast. The halfway house was due to be pulled down soon, so my daughter, Bunty, and I trawled the streets viewing everything and anything that came on the market. She had moved with me to the halfway house but we knew we needed something more permanent.

My brother Francis wasn't putting any pressure on me but I didn't want to stand in the way of his building plans, and living with my fridge outside the back door, and heating the entire house with a two bar electric fire was never meant to be a long term plan! I needed to find something in the area, cheap to maintain on my part-time nurse's budget, not too small, but definitely not too big – I was not re-visiting that horror movie. But finding that perfect in-between was proving very difficult. At least it did until the day I took a shortcut and there it was – my new home.

I knew right from the beginning it was for me. It smiled at me from its elevated position up its wonky path. It was empty following the death of its elderly owner and now it was to be sold as part of his will. One night my sister, Janet and I sneaked round the back for a nosy and there it was – a pond. My reiki house!

I couldn't wait to start bidding and I was not going to be deterred by the small fact it needed rebuilding from the inside out. I had set myself a budget with a bit to the side for work, but the crazy, Monopoly-money housing boom was raging all around me. Every phone call from the agent ate another ten thousand from my rebuilding budget. Who bids ten thousand at a time? But I hung in there, until one July afternoon I became the sale agreed owner of my beautiful dump with its wonky driveway. The formalities were to be completed in September when their solicitors completed the owner's death duties and our solicitors completed the death duties of our marriage. No winners all round. Well, maybe the solicitors.

I had only viewed the property once as I didn't need a second viewing to know it was for me. In fact, I probably didn't need a first viewing. On October 28th I turned the key into my new life, a fifties time warp, musty from its elderly occupant, but homely and warm as the sun shone through its large, front bay windows. Onward to the kitchen – it was completely un-salvageable. No paint pot could create a silk purse out of this sow's ear. But the best was yet to come, its deep peachy bathroom suite, but I think that's giving peach a bad name. Nevertheless, it was my new home, my new start and I was bubbling over with ideas and plans.

It was situated just around the corner from my halfway house so it was going to be easy to live in one while working on the other. Every evening straight in from work, hardly fed and watered, I'd put on my combats, vest top and boots and head round to demolish my new home. I pulled down, pulled out, and pulled apart anything that got in my way. Old carpets and curtains were the first casualty, to get rid of the smell. To my delight one wall-to-wall, patterned nightmare had been protecting a beautiful oak floor in the hall. But that was its only hidden treasure. Electricity, plumbing, heating, it all had to go. The building needed to be stripped bare.

I began looking for a good, new kitchen and bathroom. The ones I fell in love with were – what else? – way, way, way beyond budget. So, in order to afford them I had to economise elsewhere. I was about to become my own foreman, labourer and general dogsbody, not to mention professional skip filler!

Before the week was out we had our first skip filled with the not-to-be-salvaged kitchen. And at £155 a skip, I was determined to get my money's worth. Eight more would follow! It became a military operation. I could be seen many nights jumping on the top to make more space; how I expected my seven stone twelve pounds to make an impact, I'm not quite sure.

On one such venture my foot went through a hole. I went tumbling into a back flip worthy of an Olympic gymnast, hurtling towards the concrete ground below. Only Anthony's hand under my head saved me from a fractured skull. Right place, right time – angels at work again. I don't know who was more shaken up by this, my son or me. Skip jumping was banned after that.

There were four of us in the demolition team – Emma, John, Anthony and myself. Added to this were an electrician, and his cousin a plasterer (who moved in with us at the halfway house for two weeks and left after ten, one of them dating Emma in between!). Then there was the kitchen owner I tortured so much that he is now a great friend; a plumber, or should I say a series of plumbers, who came and went; a handyman who did handiwork because he enjoyed it; a roof man who came down from the roof to help me fill a skip; and, of course, my fairy godmothers, Sis, Janet, Katy and Claire who all mucked in.

However, when I decided to kango the terrazzo kitchen floor on a Friday, so that the team could help on Saturday to level the clods underneath, I had a mutiny on my hands. When I left them for five minutes to go round to the halfway house and make bacon sodas, they downed tools, had a whip round and called in Terry the Handyman.

A second mutiny followed. After three weeks, the demolition team were fed up eating dust and getting soaked by burst water mains, so they absconded to the hot water and comfort of their dad's. I joined the mutineers myself when my brother Bernard called one Sunday afternoon and tempted me away from my, by now, highly professional kangoing with talk of a hot meal and a warm bath. By candlelight, with a glass of wine on the side, I slid into a pampered heaven. Well, at least until I put in loads of bubble bath and switched on the Jacuzzi. I could safely say the bubbles reached the ceiling.

I couldn't find the switch to turn it off, couldn't find the edge of the bath or the plughole and as I was naked, calling my brother was out of the question. So I spent the next twenty minutes filling their shower, sink, bidet and even toilet with armloads of bubbles. Quite fun really, but not exactly the blissed-out relaxation that Sarah, my sister-in-law had intended. A ton of suds later, I finally found the plughole. I lay in the bath for five minutes and then went down for a beautiful roast dinner, my brother and Sarah quite oblivious to the mayhem I'd just caused.

*

The renovations continued. They weren't quite going to plan, but I'd set myself to be in for Christmas, so on the cold winter evenings I'd go round and work with a battery light and ice-cold water siphoned from the neighbour's outside tap. Meanwhile, my kitchen man was tearing his hair out. He said forget Christmas. It couldn't be done. But 'couldn't' wasn't a word in my vocabulary. Most times I did hold it all together but once or twice I gave way. Coming in from work to find my newly installed kitchen windows and patio doors covered in screed, I just sat on my hunkers and cried.

My volunteers had long given up and I didn't blame them, I was on my own. I was completely knackered but this mess wouldn't clean itself. Then an angel dropped by. Katy's other half popped his head in to see how things were going. One look at me and he headed off to tell Katy to get down asap, as I was at the end of reason. Then he bought some fish and chips. Fed and watered, with an emergency electric supply sorted, Katy and I washed the screed away with not-so-blue hands.

I had another crisis when the hot water tank imploded. I suppose, on the plus side, it could have been a whole lot worse if it had exploded. Or there was the night all the pipes started leaking at the million elbow joints the first plumber had inserted; or when the new water tank leaked through three floors and new plasterboard. The plumber blamed the plumbers' merchants, the plumbers' merchants blamed the plumber, while I forked out for a second tank. I didn't care who was to blame as my money was leaking through every hole in the house.

By now I'd honed my skills as foreman and labourer. I had dug out, ripped out and kangoed out every recognizable piece of the old house. It was now a blank canvas on which I could create my tapestry. I tiled, grouted, nailed down all the floorboards – only once through a pipe! I fitted eco-friendly insulation and steamed fifty years of paper from the walls, but I hope I never have the pleasure of meeting the inventor of woodchip wallpaper, as I may have something to say to him!

Determined to be in by Christmas, I had to up my game and juggle all my workmen. Who had to come before whom? Who finished after whom? Sometimes I got the order wrong but nothing major until the plasterer was waiting to plaster a ceiling. The pipes hadn't been checked, but the scaffolding had to be returned, so I told him to go ahead. Four wet patches appeared. A dose of white glug into the radiators seemed to do the trick but one area had to be cut open and repaired. Not one of my better decisions.

Nevertheless, by December I had a beautiful kitchen, two beautiful living rooms and new fireplaces, but the bathroom was posing a problem as my not to be compromised expensive sink baffled all who looked at it. Reading and re-reading the instructions failed to make sense and no one wanted to construct its wooden plinth, so I armed myself with the tools and got to work. Not perfect, but job done.

By December 22nd the last skirting board was being nailed into place while the carpet men waited on the landing. By teatime the painters' paint was drying, the new fluff was vacuumed up and I told the lads to bring round the beds as it was a Friday.

I'm not normally superstitious, but the old saying, 'a Saturday flit is a short sit' was ringing in my mind, and I didn't want to risk anything – not after all this!

So, mattress dropped on the floor, I dropped on it fully dressed. I don't remember the boys placing a throw over me, all I remember was waking up to a bright, new morning in my new home and I didn't even have to get dressed! On Saturday, John, Anthony and I bought our Christmas tree, set it up in the bare room on the bare floorboards, lit its lights and looked forward to our first Christmas in our new home.

18

Building homes

L ife was settling down. With my tool box tucked away under the stairs and the kango returned to the hire shop, it was now time to enjoy our new home, and spend time with the kids, who were slowly getting used to living between two homes with two parents who loved them loads. Now older and more independent, they decided where to stay according to what was in the fridge and what was on the menu.

Patrick and I still hadn't found any level of friendship but maybe his wounds were still too deep and raw. I had taken the life he had known and demolished it but I hoped someday he would forgive me and that he would find his own healing journey. Meanwhile Michael was taking baby steps back into my life and that was good enough for me.

Never one to sit on my hands, I was itching for a new project when Elaine whom I'd met in Lourdes suggested going away to build in Africa. Perfect! I'd learnt a lot about building over the past year and what better way to give something back than build homes for the homeless. Once I was accepted onto the Habitat for Humanity Mozambique team, I threw myself into fundraising, and before long I was digging out my passport and again heading to the airport. But this time it was as part of a team of ten strangers, not to be strangers for long.

For the next two weeks we shared a stone building with a tin roof, one plug and one toilet; mosquito nets full of holes; and plastic chairs for our wardrobe. Getting on was essential as we would be living, working, eating and sleeping twenty-four-seven together. But this wasn't hard. Laughter was often heard both on the building site and from the hostel as we grew together in friendship.

We were divided into two teams which would each try to build a roofless home a day, the thatching to be done the day after. This created a light-hearted rivalry. Cara, Catherine and I had Damien who would work the minute's silence, and Alex who at twenty-three had the strength of us three girls put together. The other team had Diane, Lyn, Beth, Nick and Alan. Evenly matched, we usually ended our days neck and neck, except on the day our supplier, the local donkey, failed to reach the site with our supplies.

By night, tired from the heat and hard work, we would all sit round a table eating the local food cooked in two large pots, playing games and having sing-songs accompanied by Nick, our very own Gareth Brooks, on his guitar. Ten adults could be heard laughing in the night while wearing post-its on their foreheads before tripping their way through dark fields to iron beds.

Tucked in under our nets and tin roof, us girls would laugh about our five star accommodation and how we didn't miss the technology of the twenty-first century. Well, at least not until the morning when a good shower would have been nice. Instead we had a cold water pipe protruding from the wall, a luxury in these parts. But when I first used it, the tap came away in my hand and a thousand ant-like creatures flooded out of the pipe over my head. Standing in a sea of insects, I couldn't move. They were swarming over me, and my Worzel Gummage hair was crawling. There was nothing else for it but to spit them out and hoke out the tap. I chose not to be the first to the shower ever again. Some girls had brought portable showers, so we would fill them up with water and leave them in the sun to heat. They were never warm enough to remove the grained in dirt, but they were wet and minus ants!

However, luxury did come our way once during the two weeks. The Irish embassy heard about our visit and decided to invite us for tea. We finished on site at lunchtime so we could all get scrubbed up for the occasion and by 3 pm we were being taken to heaven. Cold drinks, hot food, salads, fruit and soft toilet rolls. I think the ambassador couldn't understand why we all kept disappearing to the bathroom. We just stood in there with our hands under warm, clean water, sorry that we hadn't brought our bath towels with us too.

The purpose of our visit to Mozambique was to build rondavels for orphans and vulnerable children. Many had lost their parents to either malaria or Aids. The life expectancy in this land was thirty-seven years. Malaria was the main perpatrator, killing a baby under five years every thirty seconds. If this statistic occurred in the UK or the USA there would be an outcry, but in this remote part of the world, it seemed to be accepted. During our stay we managed to build fifteen homes, a dry roof for sixty children.

The following year I signed up for a second trip but this time as a team leader with Jake, a lovely gentleman and a seasoned builder. We were to build one brick construction within a week on the Mekong Delta, but in ninety-three degrees of heat this was not going to be an easy task. The team was made up of new people with the exception of Catherine who had been on the build in Mozambique. Many in the team faded from heat exhaustion and I went down with a nasty virus too. But by the weekend we managed to hang the door and welcomed its new owners.

Spending our last two days up in the forests as a treat, with a four bamboo pole raft as our only transport, maybe wasn't such a great idea after the heavy work programme. But then again, I don't think anyone in the team will ever forget the experience. We stayed overnight with a forest tribe, eating round a big fire under an Asian sky, sleeping in a stilt house on a wooden floor above their livestock; and being taken down the mountain on the backs of elephants.

Some of us took an unexpected dip in the Mekong when our raft crashed in a rapid. Elle, Nora and myself lost our possessions in the deep and nearly lost ourselves on the rocks. Wet passports, broken phones and lost cameras later, we laughed about it as we dried our sodden clothes on sticks round the campfire. Elle lined her passport, page by page, with sheets of toilet roll in a vain attempt to make it customs-worthy.

Delivered safely downstream on the elephants to civilization, we delighted in the sights and sounds of the Buddhist temples. These were filled with Lana artworks dating back to the 11th century depicting a Buddha's round face with spirals of curled hair and half closed eyes, in a seated position, one hand touching the earth to mark his enlightenment. Seated in front of these beautiful statues were young boys and men in orange robes, greeting us with a bow of the head. Shoes removed, we entered into their world of reverential silence.

Meeting Buddhist monks and being offered a Buddhist blessing made the experience complete. I knelt beside a young monk and wrote down my prayers and wishes on a small piece of paper. I then filled a silver vessel with water while the monk chanted over my head. It was a calm, gentle ceremony, in keeping with the Buddhist teachings of wisdom, peace and compassion. Twenty minutes passed in this meditative state before the monk handed me the remaining water to sprinkle over the earth outside. My blessing and prayers were complete.

Now to eat our last Thai curry and pack for home. This was to be a thirty-three hour trip through four airports: Chang Mi, Bangkok, Saudi Arabia and Dublin. But thanks to our plane nearly crash-landing on the Dublin runway, it became forty-nine hours as we were whisked away to a fifth airport. We could see Ireland, we could nearly touch Ireland – so near and yet so far! But then again, we were nearly splattered all over Ireland. So fifteen hours in a Manchester airport lobby had to be put up with while our nervous pilot slept.

Team spirit was by now in short supply. We were all tired and dirty from our long travels and some, including myself, still carried the sickness picked up on the Mekong. We tried in vain to sleep on floors and on rucksacks but these didn't quite compare to the soft beds that beckoned to us from home. That luxury wasn't to be ours for another eighteen hours.

Dublin airport! When we finally touched down, the pilot

was given a roaring round of applause from his two hundred, weary passengers. A two hour bus journey later, Jake and I finally hung up our hats. We had got the team there, built a house and had got them back safely... well, just about. The experiences we had all shared confirmed us as friends for life. As they say, in adversity you know your friends. In the Mekong, adversity created our friendships.

I came home still ill and had to hang up my hammer and my boots for a short while, but not forever. There would always be forgotten corners of the world and there would always be like-minded individuals who would travel out as strangers and return home as friends.

19

Shirley!

I was now nine years on from my cancer diagnosis and five years from my separation. I had settled into my new life and I had five charity trips behind me. The fifth one was another trip to work in the hospice, this time with daughter Emma, son John, and of course, my good friend, Seamus.

I went out to run the hospice, allowing the Sisters a much needed holiday to the coast. Seamus donned his whites and returned to his kitchen and pots of fluffy pap. Emma worked in the crèche and John worked around the grounds with the caretaker. It was a daunting task working double shifts, and being responsible for the well-being of the hospice patients as well as my two children. My brother appeared highly stressed, and the atmosphere around the hospice was more tense due to the need for increased security. Gone was the light heartedness of my first visit, but both Emma and John thrived on the experience and hoped to return in the future.

Three weeks later I returned home utterly drained, only to go and trip over my suitcase. Tearing ligaments in my ankle forced me to sit down on my backside – something I was not in the habit of doing – and take an inventory of my life. A real holiday was what I needed! A Shirley Valentine adventure!

Two months earlier I had been recalled following yet another abnormal CAT scan. Something strange had shown up on my liver and lungs. More scans needed! Feeling yet again like I was swimming through toffee, I headed home from the cancer centre to my computer and booked a solo flight to Greece. The thought in my head – life is too short for faffing about with maybes or someday...

Digging out my case from under the bed and pocketing my passport once again, I did the now familiar circuit of hugs and goodbyes. If I had any reservations about going it was not the fear of a week alone, but the worry of leaving my wonderful dad who was now fighting his own battle with this deadly disease. Hugging him tight I promised if he was in any way unwell I would be back within four hours (having taken out two insurance policies, just in case).

It is hard to watch when the rock of your life is being battered by harsh weathers. My dad, from the day he took my fat, little baby hand in his and called me his little pony, has always been there for me, the root that helped my tree grow. In childhood he taught me to tie my first shoelace, ride my first bike, swim my first length, climb my first mountain, dance my first waltz (even though there wasn't much call for it in seventies discos). But I was glad he had taught me when we shared a very special waltz on my wedding day. This time I didn't need to stand my two tiny feet on his while he burled me round the room. I was now about to stand on my own two feet, an all grown up, married lady, but it didn't stop me breaking my heart on his shoulder. When I was with him as a child I feared nothing. Not even those nuns in primary school. Or the bogey man he chased from my bedroom. Or the hard sums I couldn't add up. He made everything seem possible.

In adulthood, when cancer battered my branches he stuck them back on. When my marriage breakdown battered my branches he never judged my actions but supported me from a neutral position. And when my new tree house was collapsing around me he bought me screwdrivers to strengthen it, and a garden spade and fork to nurture its roots. Now his own branches were weakening. The cancer was taking away the power from his legs, making walking difficult. Our many, long treks over the hills of Belfast ending up on the nose of Cavehill were now a special memory to hold on to.

Only one short year ago he was a healthy man in need of no medication. Now pain control and morphine had become a part of his daily routine. Gone was his gardening, his trips to his boat and his weekends to his beloved cottage near the Mournes. The new eco car he purchased to enjoy trips around Ireland with my mum lay quiet in the driveway, only driven by my brothers as they chauffeured him to and from the hospital.

His body had slowed downed but his mind was still active. He was acutely aware of his deterioration, but continued to believe he could control it for a year or two. So when I suggested cancelling my trip he said if I didn't go, it must be because he was more ill than he thought. Damned if I stayed. Damned if I went! In the end, he made the decision for me. He packed me off with his blessing and a few pounds in my pocket... but that was my dad.

A few hours later as our plane taxied along the runway I couldn't help but smile as the dad in front pointed out to his four year old daughter.

'Look it's Ikea'!

What a pity he missed mentioning the beautiful outline of my dad's Cavehill and Napoleon's nose rising up from the river Lagan as the great, metal bird took flight.

*

My first stop on this solo journey was an overnight in London to catch up with my daughter Sam. Her new life, new man and new job! One year earlier she had taken the brave step of breaking off her engagement, cancelling her wedding plans and moving to start anew in London.

I felt a tinge of sadness when I revisited her apartment as it brought back memories of the great five days Jack and I had spent there the previous November. Ronnie Scott's, Highgate, Angel Islington... The Christmas lights were coming on all round London during our stay, but before I had mine out of their box back home, a few short weeks later, it was over. Having little in common, we had spent six months embracing our differences. Jack, the handsome boy from my past, the serious thinker of my present, but the gentle man who didn't want to hold any place in my future. He needed to be free, or maybe he just needed to be free of me.

Opening the door gently, I looked into the room and smiled sadly at the memory. Sometimes in life your heart doesn't quite keep pace with your sensible head, this was one of those moments. I boxed the memory away and closed the door on what had been.

Then I went to catch up with the madness that was my daughter in the kitchen over wine and pasta. Now a great cook she tells me. Not one for blowing her own trumpet. Meeting Max her handsome London beau and seeing her new happiness, I knew that like myself she had made the right decision, even though I might be witnessing the loss of my firstborn to this whole, new, exciting world.

20

Treasures

May shone in through London windows flooding my bedroom with sunlight. Sam and Matt had gone to their work, leaving me to breakfast on the balcony above the chimney-potted skyline. I took one last look around the apartment and checked my case and handbag because I knew when the door closed there was no going back. Wheeling my small case over London footpaths and through the underground to Gatwick, I reflected on how confident I now felt travelling alone.

Flying to a Greek island for a week – was this yet another reiki vision coming true? My home with its pond. Janet's sanctuary in Ballycastle with its marshmallow bed. Africa, holding small babies in my arms. An Amazon type river, a boat trip up the Mekong. Lourdes. So many déjà vu feelings. I slowly realised my mind had visited these special places ahead of my body, four years earlier on my sister's couch. Was this now to be the beach of my reiki where I could sit in solitude, the shackles of my life taken from me and dropped deep into the ocean? Had reiki and my grandpop given me a glimpse of what could be possible? Were my angels guiding me along this path, opening doors while closing others behind me?

*

Today, with my feet in the Aegean and my face to the sun I have reached the final chapter of this book. I came here to Kitari to finish this journey and get ready to start a new one. In 2012 it will be ten years since I felt that nondescript lump in my left breast which took me on this great adventure. Happy, sad, exhausted, exhilarated, confused, content, pushing through days filled with tears and laughter, it has been a roller coaster ride. Now, as I sit on this beautiful, Greek beach with its warm waters lapping around my feet, miles from home, miles from anyone, miles from everyone I love, I am in a good place. I am alone but not lonely. This is the final carriage in the roller coaster: to remove all the buffers of life and still be OK in the moment, in your now.

Maybe taking this trip was a way of challenging my life choices. Leaving a marriage, swimming against the tide, leaving a comfort zone, but is it a comfort to feel only a half of a whole? Today I feel whole again. I'm happy with who I am. Cancer didn't kill me, it actually gave me my life back. For too many years I was too busy to appreciate the day I was standing in; wasting time looking back over what might have been; or looking forward to what might be in the future. But cancer taught me to enjoy my here and now. Today is simple yet perfect. I watch as the water, like our life, changes with each passing second. Sometimes it carries up unwanted debris but other times it carries up the most beautiful treasures to our shore.

Over the past nine years I have so many to thank for

their treasures. My beautiful kids who have begun their own adventures in adulthood. Although I'm not needed to change their nappies, walk them to school or kiss their hurt knees better, my arms are always there to lift them to their feet. And I hope instead of giving them fish from my beach I have taught them how to fish for themselves.

My lovely parents, who in different ways have always been there for me. My mum, who found my cancer difficult to accept and my marriage break-up even harder. I broke all her rules, but five years on we agree to differ as we enjoy our love and life as mother and daughter. My dad, whose unconditional love and hugs propped me up through dark days, keeping the bogey man away. Now ill himself, it is my turn to prop him up and cherish every moment we spend together. My wonderful aunts, who gave me the gift of Lourdes and let me find sanctuary in Number Three, where I sat on the porch wrapped in the memory of my grandpop.

My Big Sis who sat with me on the beach when I felt so alone and gave me shelter in her heart and in her home and took me on wondrous adventures through reiki. My wonderful brothers, each there for me in their own way. Bernard gave me my suddy sanctuary and support. Francis held my hand beside Michael and gave me the halfway house. James gave me Africa. Martin drove me to my escape. Joseph, my little twin, who packed up my life from the Monster and with his tool belt helped me re-build my new house. John held me tight and suggested I find my lost dream. Together they built protective sandcastles around their big sister.

My friends who brought their own special gifts. Old friends,

Katy, Claire and Janet, who stayed in the roller coaster with me when it was going over the edge, helping to steady the ride, giving me a listening ear over a kitchen table, or a marshmallow bed in Ballycastle, when walking round the Cavehill wasn't enough. And Beth, Donna, Fred and the others who quietly propped me up in work when bad days had no end.

There have been new friendships with many; adventurers, blues players, charity workers, creative writers and hikers who have shared my journey; but there has been romance with none. Well, none till Jack made his brief appearance. For five years I needed to fall in love with myself. I had to re-build me without the complications of someone un-picking my handiwork. Today I like me, I think I'm OK. I am stronger because of my past, not in spite of it.

So now, alone again, I've joined a writing class and met Freda who has re-kindled the love for literature that I left behind with my Chaucer A Level books, by going to plays and discussing books and poetry over many coffees. And through a second job I've met Betty, my lovely fellow hill climber and her two friends. Together we make up Belfast's own Sex and the City foursome on our Friday nights out.

The roller coaster has stopped. The mad whirlwind of the past nine years has ended, and today I sit quietly on my Greek beach gathering up the pebbles of my life. The chipped ones haven't gone away, but I have learnt from them, and time has helped heal their scars, just like the scars on my left breast. On my dressing table back home are two letters advising me to go for two more scans next month, but each letter scares me less and less. If my cancer does return I know the pebbles on my beach will be there to support my footsteps.

What do I now want out of life?

To be happy.

To live life to the full.

To keep living my dreams.

To see my pearls flourish.

I want to laugh, to dance, to giggle, to lie on the grass with Big Sis and Janet and look at the Ballycastle stars at 3 am.

To climb Cavehill with Katy or Betty and say thank you to the sun.

To make snow angels in the snow or just stand with my feet in the Aegean.

Just like the poem given to me by Sister Adrianne on the day of my fifth cancer anniversary in the convent gardens in Africa, I want to...

Work like you don't need money
Love like you've never been hurt
And dance like no one's watching
Because happiness is the journey, not the destination.

(Writer unknown)

So, wherever I go in life I will always enjoy the journey rather than wait to be happy when I reach the destination. Today my passport is in a Greek hotel safely awaiting new journeys. If they are solo adventures I will never be alone because I will have a case load of love to take wherever I go, and I will always have my angels with me. And I don't even need to book them a room as they always sleep under my bed.